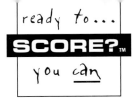

ScoreCards™ for
Ob/Gyn Sonography
A Q&A Flashcard Study System for Ob/Gyn Sonography

Traci B. Fox, EdD, RT(R), RDMS, RVT
Jefferson College of Health Professions
Thomas Jefferson University

Library of Congress Cataloging-in-Publication Data

Names: Fox, Traci B., author.

Title: ScoreCards for OB/Gyn sonography : a Q&A flashcard study system for OB/Gyn sonography / by Traci B. Fox.

Description: Pasadena, California : Davies Publishing, Inc., [2016] | Includes bibliographical references and index.

Identifiers: LCCN 2016008159 | ISBN 9780941022880 (alk. paper)

Subjects: | MESH: Pregnancy Complications--ultrasonography | Female Urogenital Diseases--ultrasonography | Pelvis--ultrasonography | Examination Questions

Classification: LCC RG107.5.U4 | NLM WQ 18.2 | DDC 618/.047543--dc23 LC

record available at http://lccn.loc.gov/2016008159

Copyright © 2017 by Davies Publishing, Inc. All rights reserved. No part of this work may be reproduced, stored in a retrieval system, or transmitted in any form or by any means, electronic or mechanical, including photocopying, scanning, and recording, without prior written permission from the publisher.

Davies Publishing, Inc.
32 South Raymond Avenue
Pasadena, California 91105-1961

Website: DaviesPublishing.com/telephone 626-792-3046

Cover and text design by Satori Design Group, Inc.

Printed in China.

ISBN 978-0-941022-88-0

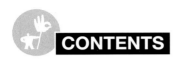

CONTENTS

How to Use *ScoreCards* v

1 OBSTETRICS 1

First Trimester 1
Gestational sac, yolk sac, embryo, ovaries, cul-de-sac, pregnancy failure, ectopic pregnancy

Second and Third Trimesters 79
Cranium, spine, heart, thorax, abdomen, extremities, fetal position

Placenta 169
Development, position, anatomy, membranes, umbilical cord, abruption, previa, masses and lesions, maturity and grading, Doppler flow studies, physiology, adherence (accreta, increta, percreta)

Assessment of Gestational Age 241
Gestational sac, embryonic size/crown-rump length, biparietal diameter, femur length, abdominal circumference, head circumference, transcerebellar measurements, binocular measurements, cephalic indices

Complications 281
Intrauterine growth restriction, multiple gestations, maternal illness, antepartum complications, fetal therapy, postpartum complications

Amniotic Fluid 355
Assessment, polyhydramnios, oligohydramnios, fetal pulmonic maturity studies

Genetic Studies 371
Maternal serum testing, amniotic fluid testing, chorionic villus sampling, dominant/recessive risk occurrence

Fetal Demise 391

Fetal Abnormalities 397
Cranial, facial, neck, neural tube, abdominal wall, thoracic, genitourinary, gastrointestinal, skeletal, cardiac, syndromes

Coexisting Disorders 621
Leiomyomas, cystic disorders, trophoblastic disease, solid/mixed masses, myometrial contraction

2 GYNECOLOGY 651

Normal Pelvic Anatomy 651
Uterus, ovaries, fallopian tubes, supporting structures, cul-de-sacs, vasculature, Doppler flow studies, gynecology-related studies

Physiology 721
Menstrual cycle, pregnancy tests, human chorionic gonadotropin, fertilization

Pediatric 755
Precocious puberty, hematometra/hematocolpos, sexual ambiguity

Infertility and Endocrinology 777
Contraception, causes, medications and treatment, ovulation induction (follicular monitoring), assisted reproductive technology (GIFT, IVF, ZIFT)

Postmenopausal 801
Anatomy, physiology, therapy, pathology

Pelvic Pathology 825
Congenital uterine malformation, uterine masses, ovarian masses, endometriosis, polycystic ovarian disease, inflammatory disease, Doppler flow studies, gynecology-related studies

Extrapelvic Pathology 899
Ascites, liver metastasis, hydronephrosis

3 PATIENT CARE, SCANNING TECHNIQUE, AND PHYSICAL PRINCIPLES 915
Review charts, communication, supine hypotensive syndrome, bioeffects, infectious disease control, scanning techniques, physical principles, artifacts

Applicaton for CME Credits 991

***ScoreCards* Cross-Referenced to the ARDMS Exam Content Outline** 1030

v

HOW TO USE *SCORECARDS*

As part of our 1-2-3 Step Ultrasound Education and Test Preparation program, *ScoreCards for Ob/Gyn Sonography* systematically prepares you to pass the Ob/Gyn Sonography exam for the Registered Diagnostic Medical Sonographer (RDMS)® credential. It also helps you to master the facts, problem-solving skills, and habits of mind that form the foundation of success not only on your registry exams but also in your career as an ultrasound professional. And it's fun.

These 495 ScoreCards cover core concepts and principles topic by topic—facts you must master to pass the Ob/Gyn exam. At the bottom of every question page is a "footer key," indicating the study topic's place within the exam coverage—from first to second/third trimester protocols, fetal anomalies to pregnancy complications, pediatric gynecology to postmenopausal pathologies—so you always know where you are and how you are doing. And at the end of the book you'll find a handy list of all these ScoreCards cross-referenced to the task-oriented ARDMS Ob/Gyn exam topics.*

*We use the last best ARDMS content outline for test preparation, updated to ensure complete coverage. The latest exam outlines from ARDMS provide a generalized categorical overview together with very specific clinical tasks, but they can miss key intermediate topics you must know to pass your exam—hence our hybrid approach to study outlines. Here you get it both ways: The table of contents reflects the key topics you need to know to pass the exam; at the end of the book, "*ScoreCards* Cross-Referenced to the ARDMS Exam Content Outline" lists the questions under the ARDMS exam outline categories that were current as of press time.

ARDMS Advanced Item Type (AIT) Questions

All questions specifically designed to prep you for the ARDMS "Advanced Item Type" (AIT) questions are identified. This is a new class of ARDMS exam question that tests practical sonographic skills by simulating hands-on clinical experience. (See "AIT Preparation Questions" at www.ARDMS.org.)

The ARDMS Ob/Gyn exam uses an Advanced Item Type called "Hotspot" questions. These items require examinees to indicate the answer to a question by using the cursor to point at or mark directly on an image. In *ScoreCards*, similar questions are identified in the question page footers as "AIT—Hotspot" questions. These flashcards ask you to indicate the label on an image that corresponds to the correct answer.

"AIT—PACSim" items are similarly marked. These highly interactive case-based Picture Archive and Communication Simulation (PACSim) questions simulate a reading station and require examinees to read a patient's clinical history, evaluate existing image(s), and complete a diagnostic ultrasound report by selecting from the options presented. Currently these items are specifically designed for reading physicians taking the Physician in Vascular Interpretation (PVI) exam; however, other specialties such as Ob/Gyn lend themselves to this type of question, so as a bonus feature we have identified such questions in the *ScoreCards* footers as well.

Finally, "AIT-SIC" (Semi-Interactive Console) items are questions that require the examinee to use a semi-interactive console to correct a problem with the image presented. These are limited to the

How to Use *ScoreCards*   vii

Sonography Principles and Instrumentation (SPI) examination. They do not appear in the Ob/Gyn specialty exam and are therefore not included among these Ob/Gyn ScoreCards.

Tips for Maximizing Your Learning

Here are some tips for maximizing the value of the *ScoreCards* system:

Take it with you. The *ScoreCards* study system is designed to be portable. Use it on breaks or between patients. You can review a dozen question/answer items in five minutes.

Study, test yourself, review. As you study for the ARDMS specialty exam in Ob/Gyn sonography, *ScoreCards* drills you on key facts and figures, it tests your knowledge of those facts in practical situations, and it provides clear explanations and references for further study. Each Q&A card is keyed to the table of contents. You always know where you are, how you are doing, and how important the topic is to your overall success on the exam.

Triangulate on your target. By itself, the *ScoreCards* study system is a powerful, convenient, and fun way of learning and testing yourself. It is especially effective when used with *Ob/Gyn Sonography: An Illustrated Review* (Step 1: review text) and *Ob/Gyn Sonography Review* (Step 2: mock examination). Just as each ScoreCard tells you which study topic it covers, it also indicates exactly where you can find further information about the subject, often in the Step 1 review text. So do the Davies mock examinations. This integrated, systematic strategy triangulates on your target—exam and career success!

viii   How to Use *ScoreCards*

Shuffle it! After using the flipcard format for a while, consider removing the spiral binding and mixing up the cards to vary the order in which they challenge you.

Earn CME credit. The *ScoreCards* study system is an SDMS-approved CME activity that can help meet the CME requirements necessary to maintain your registry status once you pass your exams. Use the CME application that follows the last question in this book. You may use the CME application anywhere, anytime, at your convenience.

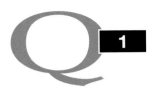

Q1

What is the earliest sonographic sign of a pregnancy?

a. double bleb sign
b. double sac sign
c. yolk sac
d. decidual thickening

Obstetrics / First Trimester

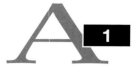

D. Decidual thickening.

Thickening of the endometrium is an early sign of pregnancy. Thickening does not always confirm an intrauterine pregnancy (IUP), as the uterine lining will increase in size in the presence of an ectopic pregnancy as well. Follow-up ultrasound and serial beta-hCG values must be obtained to confirm an IUP.

▶ Baun J: *Ob/Gyn Sonography: An Illustrated Review*. Pasadena, CA, Davies Publishing, 2016, p 8.

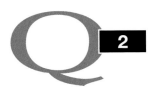

A normal gestational sac grows at the rate of:

a. 0.5 mm per day
b. 1.1 mm per day
c. 1.5 mm per day
d. 2.1 mm per day

Obstetrics / First Trimester

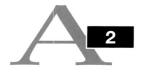

B. 1.1 mm per day.

> The normal gestational sac has a growth rate of approximately 1.1 mm per day. Inadequate gestational sac growth may be a predictor of pregnancy failure.

▶ Baun J: *Ob/Gyn Sonography: An Illustrated Review*. Pasadena, CA, Davies Publishing, 2016, p 14.

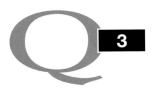

3

What is the term for the sonographic appearance of a small fluid-filled sac contained within the decidua at approximately 4.0–4.5 menstrual weeks?

a. double bleb sign
b. double sac sign
c. intradecidual sign
d. pseudogestational sac sign

Obstetrics / First Trimester

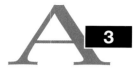

C. Intradecidual sign.

The intradecidual sign represents the very early gestational sac. This sign is seen prior to the appearance of the secondary yolk sac.

▶ Baun J: *Ob/Gyn Sonography: An Illustrated Review*. Pasadena, CA, Davies Publishing, 2016, p 9.

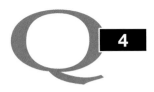

Q 4

When can you first identify a gestational sac using endovaginal sonography?

a. 4–5 menstrual weeks
b. 2–3 menstrual weeks
c. 5–6 menstrual weeks
d. 6–7 menstrual weeks

Obstetrics / First Trimester

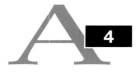

A. 4–5 menstrual weeks.

The gestational sac can be seen as early as 4–5 menstrual weeks, but an intrauterine pregnancy (IUP) cannot be confirmed until the secondary yolk sac is seen, typically at about 5–6 menstrual weeks.

▶ Baun J: *Ob/Gyn Sonography: An Illustrated Review*. Pasadena, CA, Davies Publishing, 2016, p 8.
▶ Gill KA: Gynecology. In Gill KA: *Ultrasound in Obstetrics and Gynecology: A Practitioner's Guide*. Pasadena, CA, Davies Publishing, 2014, p 97.

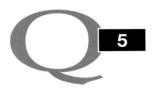 5

What term describes the echogenic ring formed by the decidua parietalis and decidua capsularis?

a. double bleb sign
b. intradecidual sign
c. double decidual sac sign
d. pseudogestational sac sign

Obstetrics / First Trimester

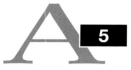

C. Double decidual sac sign.

The *decidua parietalis* (also called the *decidua vera*) and the *decidua capsularis* can be visualized together at 5.5–6.0 menstrual weeks and indicate the presence of a pregnancy. Their appearance together is known as the *double decidual sac sign* or *double decidual ring sign*.

- Baun J: *Ob/Gyn Sonography: An Illustrated Review*. Pasadena, CA, Davies Publishing, 2016, p 10.
- Sliman MH, Gill KA: The first trimester. In Gill KA: *Ultrasound in Obstetrics and Gynecology: A Practitioner's Guide*. Pasadena, CA, Davies Publishing, 2014, pp 95–96.

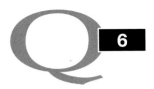

What does the appearance of an anechoic cystic structure in the endometrial canal most likely indicate?

a. early intrauterine pregnancy
b. pseudosac
c. complete abortion
d. molar pregnancy

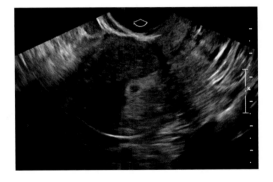

Obstetrics / First Trimester

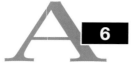

B. Pseudosac.

A cystic structure seen in the central endometrium is suspicious for a pseudosac from an ectopic pregnancy. An intrauterine pregnancy (IUP) is typically eccentrically located, not centrally located, in the endometrium. These findings need to be considered along with the patient's clinical history.

▶ Sliman MH, Gill KA: The first trimester. In Gill KA: *Ultrasound in Obstetrics and Gynecology: A Practitioner's Guide*. Pasadena, CA, Davies Publishing, 2014, pp 94, 97, 109.

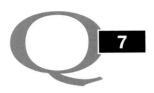

The structure seen in this sonographic image (arrow) most likely represents the:

a. primary yolk sac
b. amnion
c. chorion
d. secondary yolk sac

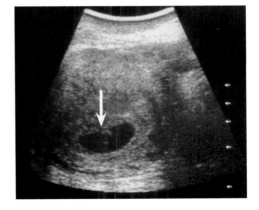

Obstetrics / First Trimester / AIT—Hotspot

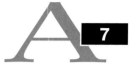

D. Secondary yolk sac.

The primary yolk sac, which cannot be visualized by ultrasound, regresses at 4 menstrual weeks and the secondary yolk sac replaces it. The secondary yolk sac is typically seen in the gestational sac by 5.5 menstrual weeks.

- Baun J: *Ob/Gyn Sonography: An Illustrated Review*. Pasadena, CA, Davies Publishing, 2016, p 10.
- Sliman MH, Gill KA: The first trimester. In Gill KA: *Ultrasound in Obstetrics and Gynecology: A Practitioner's Guide*. Pasadena, CA, Davies Publishing, 2014, p 94.

In a normal pregnancy, the yolk sac will always be visualized when the mean sac diameter is:

a. ≥5.0 mm
b. ≥8.0 mm
c. ≥6.0 mm
d. ≥7.0 mm

Obstetrics / First Trimester

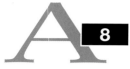

B. ≥8.0 mm.

In a normal pregnancy, using a transvaginal approach, the secondary yolk sac can sometimes be visualized by 5 weeks, when mean sac diameter (MSD) is 5 mm, but can always be visualized by 5.5 menstrual weeks, when the MSD is 8 mm.

▶ Baun J: *Ob/Gyn Sonography: An Illustrated Review*. Pasadena, CA, Davies Publishing, 2016, p 10.

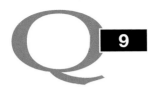

Identify the abnormal finding on this image.

a. embryonic hydrocephalus
b. abdominal wall defect
c. abnormal yolk sac
d. molar changes in placenta

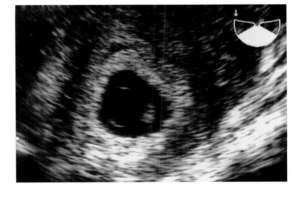

Obstetrics / First Trimester

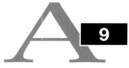

C. Abnormal yolk sac.

The gestational sac and embryo appear normal for the stage of pregnancy; however, the yolk sac should not be so large in relation to the embryonic pole.

▶ Baun J: *Ob/Gyn Sonography: An Illustrated Review*. Pasadena, CA, Davies Publishing, 2016, p 14.
▶ Sliman MH, Gill KA: The first trimester. In Gill KA: *Ultrasound in Obstetrics and Gynecology: A Practitioner's Guide*. Pasadena, CA, Davies Publishing, 2014, pp 94–95.

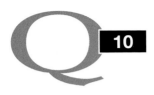

Which sonographic finding indicates an abnormal pregnancy?

a. embryo with calcified yolk sac
b. defined double decidual ring around the intrauterine gestational sac
c. round or oval gestational sac within the uterus
d. double sac sign within an intrauterine gestational sac

Obstetrics / First Trimester

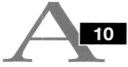

A. Embryo with calcified yolk sac.

Secondary yolk sacs should be round and well defined. Those that are flat, irregular in shape, calcified, enlarged, absent, or solid in appearance would indicate an abnormal pregnancy with the possibility of impending abortion.

- Baun J: *Ob/Gyn Sonography: An Illustrated Review*. Pasadena, CA, Davies Publishing, 2016, p 14.
- Sliman MH, Gill KA: The first trimester. In Gill KA: *Ultrasound in Obstetrics and Gynecology: A Practitioner's Guide*. Pasadena, CA, Davies Publishing, 2014, p 94.

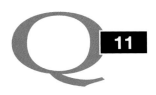 11

Which yolk sac finding is associated with a good pregnancy outcome?

a. <2 mm at 8–10 weeks
b. round shape
c. irregular echogenic borders
d. >6 mm in diameter

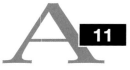

B. Round shape.

The normal yolk sac is round and measures between 2 mm and 6 mm in diameter. A small, absent, misshapen, or calcified yolk sac suggests a poor prognosis.

- Baun J: *Ob/Gyn Sonography: An Illustrated Review*. Pasadena, CA, Davies Publishing, 2016, pp 10, 14.
- Sliman MH, Gill KA: The first trimester. In Gill KA: *Ultrasound in Obstetrics and Gynecology: A Practitioner's Guide*. Pasadena, CA, Davies Publishing, 2014, p 94.

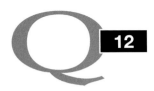

Q 12

With transvaginal ultrasound, a fetal pole with cardiac motion should always be identifiable by the time the mean sac diameter (MSD) is:

a. 16 mm

b. 20 mm

c. 25 mm

d. 30 mm

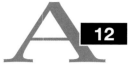

A. 16 mm.

When interrogating a normal pregnancy with transvaginal sonography, you should be able to identify a fetal pole with a heartbeat when the mean sac diameter (MSD) is greater than or equal to 16 mm. Transabdominally, cardiac motion should be visualized when the MSD is greater than or equal to 25 mm.

- Baun J: *Ob/Gyn Sonography: An Illustrated Review*. Pasadena, CA, Davies Publishing, 2016, pp 10–12.
- Rodriguez J, Gill KA: Anomalies associated with oligohydramnios. In Gill KA: *Ultrasound in Obstetrics and Gynecology: A Practitioner's Guide*. Pasadena, CA, Davies Publishing, 2014, p 99.

How does conceptual age relate to menstrual age?

a. Conceptual age is 14 days less than menstrual age.
b. Conceptual age is 7 days greater than menstrual age.
c. Conceptual age is 14 days greater than menstrual age.
d. Conceptual age is 7 days less than menstrual age.

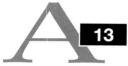

A. Conceptual age is 14 days less than menstrual age.

Fertilization of the ovum (conception) is said to occur around day 14 of the menstrual cycle. However, menstrual age is calculated using the first day of the last menstrual period (LMP), which is typically 14 days before the date of conception. Therefore, at the moment of conception, the pregnancy is already two weeks old by LMP.

▶ Baun J: *Ob/Gyn Sonography: An Illustrated Review*. Pasadena, CA, Davies Publishing, 2016, p 5.

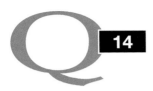

The arrow in this image of a 10-week fetus points to:

a. gastroschisis
b. omphalocele
c. umbilical vein thrombosis
d. normal embryonic midgut herniation

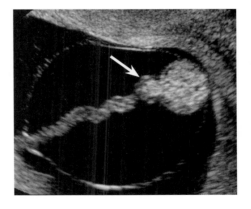

Obstetrics / First Trimester / AIT—Hotspot

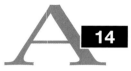

D. Normal embryonic midgut herniation.

Physiologic herniation of the bowel is part of a normal process of bowel growth and rotation and is normally visualized between 8 and 12 menstrual weeks. By 12 weeks the normal bowel should have regressed into the abdomen. Any bowel seen in the base of the umbilical cord after 12 weeks should be considered an omphalocele until proven otherwise.

- Baun J: *Ob/Gyn Sonography: An Illustrated Review*. Pasadena, CA, Davies Publishing, 2016, p 12.
- Sliman MH, Gill KA: The first trimester. In Gill KA: *Ultrasound in Obstetrics and Gynecology: A Practitioner's Guide*. Pasadena, CA, Davies Publishing, 2014, p 100.

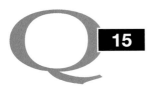

The arrow in this image points to:

a. hydrocephalus
b. cisterna magna
c. embryonic rhombencephalon
d. nuchal translucency

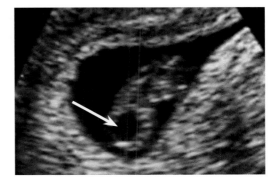

Obstetrics / First Trimester / AIT—Hotspot

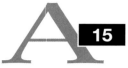

C. Embryonic rhombencephalon.

>   The rhombencephalon is a primitive hindbrain structure that appears as a fluid-filled space. It is a normal structure in the embryo.

▶ Baun J: *Ob/Gyn Sonography: An Illustrated Review*. Pasadena, CA, Davies Publishing, 2016, p 13.

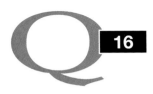

16

Embryonic cardiac activity may be visualized when the crown-rump length (CRL) is approximately:

a. 1–3 mm
b. 2–4 mm
c. 3–5 mm
d. 4–6 mm

Obstetrics / First Trimester

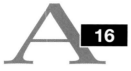

B. 2–4 mm.

Embryonic cardiac activity may be seen as early as 5 weeks transvaginally, which corresponds to a CRL of 2–4 mm. It is possible to see embryonic cardiac activity adjacent to the yolk sac even before the CRL is visualized. If cardiac activity is not seen with a CRL of 5 mm or greater, nonviability should be suspected.

▶ Baun J: *Ob/Gyn Sonography: An Illustrated Review*. Pasadena, CA, Davies Publishing, 2016, p 10.

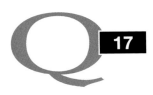

What is the name of the conceptus when it implants in the uterine lining?

a. zygote
b. morula
c. blastocyst
d. yolk sac

Obstetrics / First Trimester

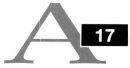

C. Blastocyst.

> The fertilized ovum is called the *zygote*. The zygote goes on to form the *morula*, which then becomes the *blastocyst*. It is the blastocyst that implants into the uterine lining.

- Baun J: *Ob/Gyn Sonography: An Illustrated Review*. Pasadena, CA, Davies Publishing, 2016, p 6.
- Sliman MH, Gill KA: The first trimester. In Gill KA: *Ultrasound in Obstetrics and Gynecology: A Practitioner's Guide*. Pasadena, CA, Davies Publishing, 2014, p 91.

Q 18

The fluid-filled cavity in which the embryo develops is the:

a. amniotic cavity
b. yolk sac
c. blastocyst
d. chorionic cavity

Obstetrics / First Trimester

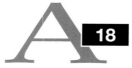

A. Amniotic cavity.

The amniotic cavity grows as the ventral folding of the embryo occurs at about menstrual week 5. The amniotic cavity will house the developing embryo and will continue to expand until it reaches the chorionic cavity.

- Ballao LA: Sonembryology. In AIUM: *Update in Ob/Gyn Ultrasound*. Laurel, NJ, American Institute of Ultrasound in Medicine, 1996, pp 1–10.
- Baun J: *Ob/Gyn Sonography: An Illustrated Review*. Pasadena, CA, Davies Publishing, 2016, pp 6–7.

Implantation occurs approximately how many days after the beginning of the last menstrual period?

a. 17 to 18 days
b. 19 to 20 days
c. 21 to 22 days
d. 23 to 24 days

Obstetrics / First Trimester

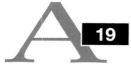

C. 21 to 22 days.

Approximately three weeks after the first day of the last menstrual period (LMP), the blastocyst implants into the endometrium. Hence implantation occurs at approximately 3 weeks' menstrual age, or a conceptual age of approximately 1 week.

- Baun J: *Ob/Gyn Sonography: An Illustrated Review*. Pasadena, CA, Davies Publishing, 2016, p 7.
- Callen PW: *Ultrasonography in Obstetrics and Gynecology*, 5th edition. Philadelphia, Elsevier, 2008, pp 184–185.

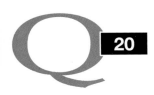

How many weeks after conception does the embryo become a fetus?

a. 6
b. 10
c. 8
d. 12

Obstetrics / First Trimester

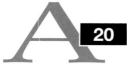

C. 8.

All major organ systems have formed by 8 weeks from conception, or 10 weeks' menstrual age—marking the transition from embryo to fetus.

- Baun J: *Ob/Gyn Sonography: An Illustrated Review*. Pasadena, CA, Davies Publishing, 2016, p 4.
- Sliman MH, Gill KA: The first trimester. In Gill KA: *Ultrasound in Obstetrics and Gynecology: A Practitioner's Guide*. Pasadena, CA, Davies Publishing, 2014, p 90.

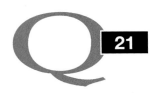

Q 21

Which hormone does the corpus luteum produce?

a. progesterone
b. follicle-stimulating hormone
c. luteinizing hormone
d. estradiol

Obstetrics / First Trimester

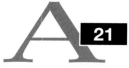

A. Progesterone.

The corpus luteum produces progesterone, necessary to sustain the developing pregnancy. The placenta takes over this function after approximately 8 weeks.

- Baun J: *Ob/Gyn Sonography: An Illustrated Review*. Pasadena, CA, Davies Publishing, 2016, p 16.
- Cunningham FG, Leveno KJ, Bloom SL, et al: *Williams Obstetrics*, 24th edition. New York, McGraw-Hill, 2014, p 107.

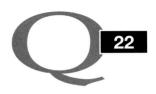

Q 22

Corpus luteum cysts of pregnancy typically regress by:

a. 6–8 weeks
b. 8–10 weeks
c. 12–16 weeks
d. 10–12 weeks

Obstetrics / First Trimester

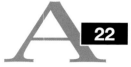

C. 12–16 weeks.

Although it may regress as early as 6–8 weeks, the corpus luteum cyst of pregnancy should be resolved by 12–16 weeks (according to some authors, up to 18–20 weeks).

- Baun J: *Ob/Gyn Sonography: An Illustrated Review*. Pasadena, CA, Davies Publishing, 2016, p 16.
- Gill KA: Gynecology. In Gill KA: *Ultrasound in Obstetrics and Gynecology: A Practitioner's Guide*. Pasadena, CA, Davies Publishing, 2014, p 58.
- Morgan MA, Jones J: Corpus luteum. Radiopaedia. Available at http://radiopaedia.org/articles/corpus-luteum.

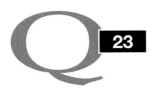

The fluid collection in this image is located in the:

a. space of Retzius
b. anterior cul-de-sac
c. Morison's pouch
d. posterior cul-de-sac

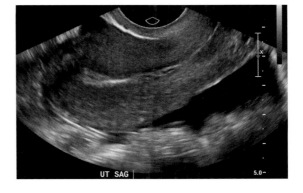

Obstetrics / First Trimester / AIT—Hotspot

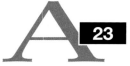

D. Posterior cul-de-sac.

The posterior cul-de-sac is also known as the *pouch of Douglas* or *rectouterine space*. It is a common place for free fluid to collect in a supine patient.

▶ Baun J: *Ob/Gyn Sonography: An Illustrated Review*. Pasadena, CA, Davies Publishing, 2016, pp 19, 355.
▶ Gill KA: Gynecology. In Gill KA: *Ultrasound in Obstetrics and Gynecology: A Practitioner's Guide*. Pasadena, CA, Davies Publishing, 2014, pp 31, 32, 34.

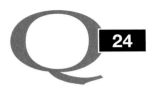

What is the arrow pointing to in this image?

a. fluid in the anterior cul-de-sac
b. fluid in the posterior cul-de-sac
c. fluid in the endometrial cavity
d. fluid in the space of Retzius

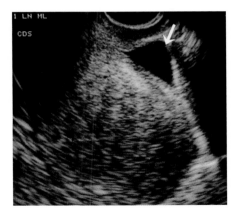

Obstetrics / First Trimester / AIT—Hotspot

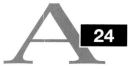

B. Fluid in the posterior cul-de-sac.

Because the uterus is retroflexed, this fluid is in the posterior cul-de-sac. The bladder, if seen, would be at the left upper corner of the image, as would the anterior cul-de-sac.

- Baun J: *Ob/Gyn Sonography: An Illustrated Review*. Pasadena, CA, Davies Publishing, 2016, p 355.
- Gill KA: *Ultrasound in Obstetrics and Gynecology: A Practitioner's Guide*. Pasadena, CA, Davies Publishing, 2014, pp 21, 22.

In what pelvic space will the ovaries never be visualized?

a. adnexa
b. ovarian fossa
c. anterior cul-de-sac
d. posterior cul-de-sac

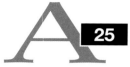

C. Anterior cul-de-sac.

The anterior cul-de-sac, which is the space between the uterus and the bladder, is also called the *uterovesical space*. The ovaries are not found in this location.

▶ Gill KA: Gynecology. In Gill KA: *Ultrasound in Obstetrics and Gynecology: A Practitioner's Guide*. Pasadena, CA, Davies Publishing, 2014, p 31.

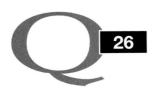
26

The sonographic demonstration of cervical dilatation in the first trimester suggests:

a. spontaneous abortion
b. inevitable abortion
c. incomplete abortion
d. threatened abortion

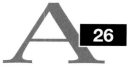

B. Inevitable abortion.

A dilated cervix in the first or early second trimester is a sign of an inevitable or impending abortion. The embryo/fetus may be alive despite the low position in the sac, but the pregnancy is going to be lost.

▶ Sliman MH, Gill KA: The first trimester. In Gill KA: *Ultrasound in Obstetrics and Gynecology: A Practitioner's Guide*. Pasadena, CA, Davies Publishing, 2014, p 103.

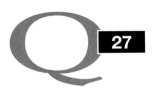

27

What is the term for physiologic termination of pregnancy prior to 20 weeks' gestation?

a. spontaneous abortion
b. blighted ovum
c. anembryonic pregnancy
d. therapeutic abortion

Obstetrics / First Trimester

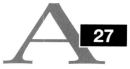

A. Spontaneous abortion.

Spontaneous abortion (SAB)—commonly referred to as a *miscarriage*—is the physiologic termination of pregnancy prior to 20 weeks' gestation. Approximately 12% of all pregnancies end in spontaneous abortion, with 75% occurring before the 16th week. Spontaneous abortions may be complete or incomplete.

▶ Baun J: *Ob/Gyn Sonography: An Illustrated Review*. Pasadena, CA, Davies Publishing, 2016, pp 15–17.

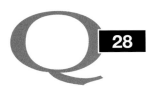

What is the finding in this 9-week gestation with vaginal bleeding?

a. incomplete abortion
b. spontaneous abortion
c. threatened abortion
d. inevitable abortion

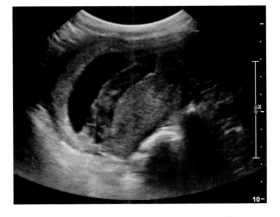

Obstetrics / First Trimester

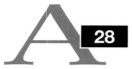

C. Threatened abortion.

This image reveals a gestational sac with a subchorionic hemorrhage. A patient who presents with vaginal bleeding at less than 20 weeks is said to have a threatened abortion.

- Baun J: *Ob/Gyn Sonography: An Illustrated Review*. Pasadena, CA, Davies Publishing, 2016, p 16.
- Raatz Stephenson S (ed): *Diagnostic Medical Sonography: Obstetrics and Gynecology*, 3rd edition. Baltimore, Lippincott Williams & Wilkins, 2012, ch 14.

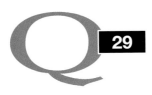

Q 29

Your patient has an intact gestational sac measuring more than 25 mm transabdominally in the endometrial cavity, but no embryo is visualized within the sac. What is this condition called?

a. complete spontaneous abortion
b. anembryonic pregnancy
c. incomplete abortion
d. fetal demise

Obstetrics / First Trimester

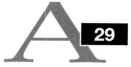

B. Anembryonic pregnancy.

The diagnosis of anembryonic pregnancy (formerly known as *blighted ovum*) can be made when no embryo is seen and the mean sac diameter (MSD) is greater than 25 mm transabdominally or greater than 18 mm transvaginally.

▶ Baun J: *Ob/Gyn Sonography: An Illustrated Review*. Pasadena, CA, Davies Publishing, 2016, p 16.

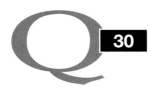

In this patient with an irregular gestational sac and no fetal heart motion, what is the most likely diagnosis?

a. ectopic pregnancy
b. anembryonic pregnancy
c. threatened abortion
d. embryonic demise

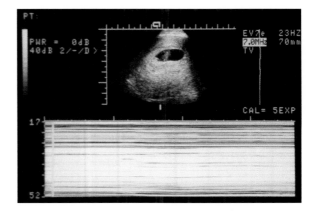

Obstetrics / First Trimester

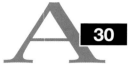

D. Embryonic demise.

This image demonstrates embryonic demise, or incomplete abortion. The embryo is noted in the uterine cavity but no heart motion was detected. An ectopic pregnancy would be located outside the uterus, an anembryonic pregnancy or blighted ovum would reveal a large, empty gestational sac, and *threatened abortion* is a clinical term used whenever a pregnant patient has first trimester bleeding.

▶ Baun J: *Ob/Gyn Sonography: An Illustrated Review*. Pasadena, CA, Davies Publishing, 2016, p 15.
▶ Sliman MH, Gill KA: The first trimester. In Gill KA: *Ultrasound in Obstetrics and Gynecology: A Practitioner's Guide*. Pasadena, CA, Davies Publishing, 2014, p 104.

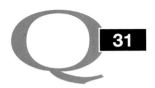

This patient presents with bleeding and cramping. Her pregnancy test is weakly positive. Three days prior, a living IUP was documented in the uterus. This transvaginal image suggests:

a. incomplete abortion
b. ectopic pregnancy
c. normal intrauterine pregnancy
d. pseudocyesis

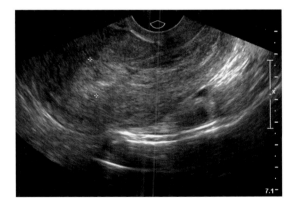

Obstetrics / First Trimester / AIT—PACSim

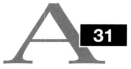

A. Incomplete abortion.

Given the patient's history, the most likely diagnosis is incomplete abortion. The uterus contains tissue but shows nothing that represents a normal pregnancy. An ectopic pregnancy or pseudocyesis would present with an empty uterus. Molar tissue usually shows multiple cystic areas representative of hydropic changes within the placenta.

- Baun J: *Ob/Gyn Sonography: An Illustrated Review*. Pasadena, CA, Davies Publishing, 2016, p 15.
- Sliman MH, Gill KA: The first trimester. In Gill KA: *Ultrasound in Obstetrics and Gynecology: A Practitioner's Guide*. Pasadena, CA, Davies Publishing, 2014, pp 102–103.

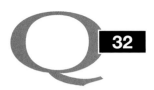

This patient presented with bleeding in the first trimester. What is the probable finding?

a. spontaneous abortion
b. complete abortion
c. inevitable abortion
d. threatened abortion

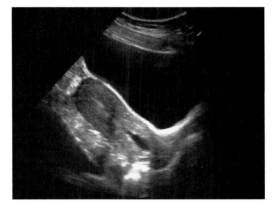

Obstetrics / First Trimester

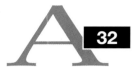

C. Inevitable abortion.

This image demonstrates a sac low in the uterus, consistent with inevitable, or impending, abortion. A threatened abortion would appear as a subchorionic hemorrhage. A complete abortion (which is one type of spontaneous abortion) would appear as an empty uterus.

▶ Sliman MH, Gill KA: The first trimester. In Gill KA: *Ultrasound in Obstetrics and Gynecology: A Practitioner's Guide*. Pasadena, CA, Davies Publishing, 2014, pp 103–104.

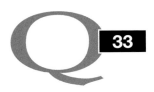

Implantation of a conceptus anywhere outside the central portion of the endometrial cavity is called:

a. incomplete abortion
b. missed abortion
c. blighted ovum
d. ectopic pregnancy

Obstetrics / First Trimester

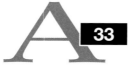

D. Ectopic pregnancy.

An ectopic pregnancy is one that is not normally implanted in the uterus. An ectopic pregnancy can occur anywhere but most commonly occurs in the fallopian tube.

▶ Baun J: *Ob/Gyn Sonography: An Illustrated Review*. Pasadena, CA, Davies Publishing, 2016, p 17.

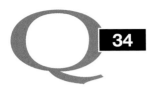

A patient presents with a serum beta-hCG titer at discriminatory levels. She complains of lower-quadrant pain and vaginal spotting. Sonographic examination of the adnexa produces the results shown in this image. What is the most likely diagnosis?

a. complete abortion
b. invasive mole
c. ectopic pregnancy
d. hydatidiform mole

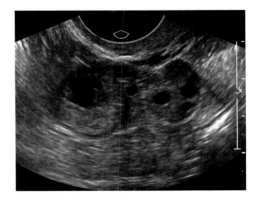

Obstetrics / First Trimester / AIT—PACSim

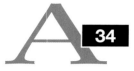

C. Ectopic pregnancy.

This patient has a positive beta-hCG titer, pain, bleeding, and an adnexal mass. This is presumed to be an ectopic pregnancy. Remember that even in a patient with an intrauterine pregnancy, there is the possibility of a coexisting ectopic pregnancy. When this occurs it is called a *heterotopic pregnancy.*

▶ Baun J: *Ob/Gyn Sonography: An Illustrated Review*. Pasadena, CA, Davies Publishing, 2016, pp 17–20.

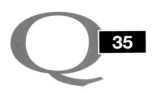

Q 35

Of the following, which is the most common site for an ectopic pregnancy?

a. cornua
b. cervix
c. abdomen
d. ampulla

Obstetrics / First Trimester

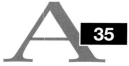

D. Ampulla.

The ampullary portion of the fallopian tube is the most common site of ectopic pregnancies. All of the other choices can be sites of ectopic pregnancy but are considered much less common.

- Baun J: *Ob/Gyn Sonography: An Illustrated Review*. Pasadena, CA, Davies Publishing, 2016, p 18.
- Sliman MH, Gill KA: The first trimester. In Gill KA: *Ultrasound in Obstetrics and Gynecology: A Practitioner's Guide*. Pasadena, CA, Davies Publishing, 2014, pp 105–106.

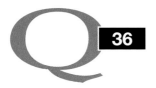

Your patient presents with a beta-hCG level of 5,730 mlU/ml, pain in the right lower quadrant, and bright red spotting. This history and the transverse image shown here suggest that the most likely diagnosis is:

a. hemorrhagic corpus luteum
b. threatened abortion
c. intrauterine pregnancy
d. ectopic pregnancy

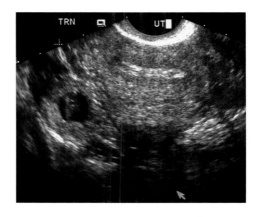

Obstetrics / First Trimester / AIT—PACSim

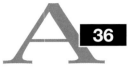

D. Ectopic pregnancy.

The image shows the uterus to be empty, which rules out threatened abortion and trophoblastic disease. With a beta-hCG level of 5,730 mIU/ml, you should be able to see an intrauterine gestational sac. There is a mass in the right adnexa that could be a hemorrhagic corpus luteum, but this patient has the classic triad of symptoms for ectopic pregnancy. Any patient with a positive beta-hCG titer and an empty uterus—with or without an adnexal mass—should be considered for a possible ectopic pregnancy until it is proven otherwise.

▶ Baun J: *Ob/Gyn Sonography: An Illustrated Review*. Pasadena, CA, Davies Publishing, 2016, pp 17–20.
▶ Sliman MH, Gill KA: The first trimester. In Gill KA: *Ultrasound in Obstetrics and Gynecology: A Practitioner's Guide*. Pasadena, CA, Davies Publishing, 2014, pp 105–111.

Q 37

Heterotopic pregnancy refers to:

a. an irregular sac-like structure in the endometrium
b. a simultaneous intra- and extrauterine pregnancy
c. an irregular sac-like structure in the adnexa
d. an abdominal pregnancy

Obstetrics / First Trimester

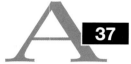

B. A simultaneous intra- and extrauterine pregnancy.

Heterotopic pregnancy occurs when both an intrauterine pregnancy (IUP) and a coexisting ectopic pregnancy occur at the same time. Remember: The presence of an IUP does not rule out ectopic pregnancy. The adnexa must be scanned thoroughly.

▶ Baun J: *Ob/Gyn Sonography: An Illustrated Review*. Pasadena, CA, Davies Publishing, 2016, pp 14, 18, 19.
▶ Sliman MH, Gill KA: The first trimester. In Gill KA: *Ultrasound in Obstetrics and Gynecology: A Practitioner's Guide*. Pasadena, CA, Davies Publishing, 2014, p 110.

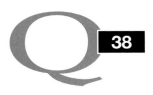

A noninvasive treatment for ectopic pregnancy is:

a. dilatation and curettage
b. culdocentesis
c. laparotomy
d. methotrexate therapy

Obstetrics / First Trimester

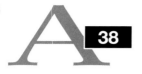

D. Methotrexate therapy.

Methotrexate is a pharmaceutical, nonsurgical treatment for ectopic pregnancy. Specific criteria must be met for patients to be treated with methotrexate, and these criteria may vary by institution. Surgery is usually performed in the presence of a suspected ruptured ectopic pregnancy.

- Callen PW: *Ultrasonography in Obstetrics and Gynecology*, 5th edition. Philadelphia, Elsevier, 2008, p 1042.
- Stearns T: Effects of maternal disease on pregnancy. In Raatz Stephenson S (ed): *Diagnostic Medical Sonography: Obstetrics and Gynecology*, 3rd edition. Philadelphia, Lippincott Williams & Wilkins, 2012, ch 29.

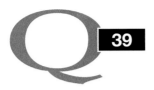

This image is from a patient whose last normal menstrual period was 8 weeks before and whose beta-hCG level had plateaued. What does this sonogram reveal?

a. right interstitial ectopic pregnancy
b. normal intrauterine pregnancy in the corpus
c. right ampullary tube ectopic pregnancy
d. right ovarian ectopic pregnancy

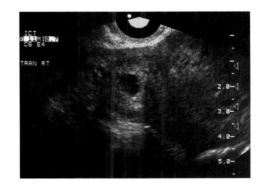

Obstetrics / First Trimester / AIT—PACSim

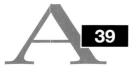

A. Right interstitial ectopic pregnancy.

Interstitial ectopic pregnancies are dangerous because of the vast blood supply in this location and because interstitial ectopic pregnancies—unlike tubal ectopic pregnancies—typically go unnoticed until later in gestation. Rupture of an interstitial pregnancy can lead to massive blood loss and death from exsanguination.

▶ Sliman MH, Gill KA: The first trimester. In Gill KA: *Ultrasound in Obstetrics and Gynecology: A Practitioner's Guide*. Pasadena, CA, Davies Publishing, 2014, pp 109–110.

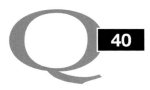

The arrows in this image are pointing to:

a. thalami
b. cerebellum
c. ventricles
d. cisterna magna

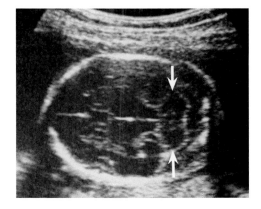

Obstetrics / Second and Third Trimesters / AIT—Hotspot

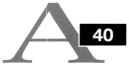

B. Cerebellum.

▶ Baun J: *Ob/Gyn Sonography: An Illustrated Review*. Pasadena, CA, Davies Publishing, 2016, p 73.

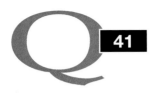 41

In the fetal brain, the highly vascularized structure lying along the floor of both lateral ventricles and extending along the roof of the third ventricle is the:

a. choroid plexus
b. cavum septi pellucidi
c. falx cerebri
d. corpus callosum

Obstetrics / Second and Third Trimesters

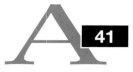

A. Choroid plexus.

The choroid plexus, which is the markedly echogenic structure seen within the fetal brain, produces cerebrospinal fluid (CSF) that fills the ventricles. It is located mainly in the atria of the lateral ventricles and the roof of the third ventricle.

▶ Baun J: *Ob/Gyn Sonography: An Illustrated Review*. Pasadena, CA, Davies Publishing, 2016, pp 113, 115.

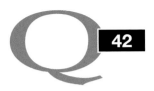

Q 42

Which of the following cranial structures serves as the landmark for locating the atria of the lateral ventricles?

a. cavum septi pellucidi
b. corpus callosum
c. cisterna magna
d. choroid plexus

Obstetrics / Second and Third Trimesters

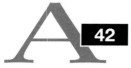

D. Choroid plexus.

The choroid plexus is located between the medial and lateral walls of the atria of the lateral ventricles of the brain.

- Baun J: *Ob/Gyn Sonography: An Illustrated Review*. Pasadena, CA, Davies Publishing, 2016, pp 115–116.
- Rodriguez J, Gill KA: The second and third trimesters: basic and targeted scans. In Gill KA: *Ultrasound in Obstetrics and Gynecology: A Practitioner's Guide*. Pasadena, CA, Davies Publishing, 2014, p 125.

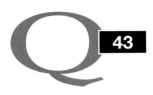**43**

What are the normal measurements for the lateral ventricle of the fetal brain?

a. 1 mm in the largest dimension transversely
b. 10 mm in the largest dimension longitudinally
c. 1 cm in the largest dimension transversely
d. 1 cm in the largest dimension longitudinally

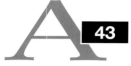

C. 1 cm in the largest dimension transversely.

> Baun J: *Ob/Gyn Sonography: An Illustrated Review*. Pasadena, CA, Davies Publishing, 2016, p 113.

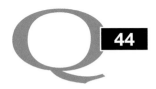

What does the structure in the posterior section of the fetal head represent in this image?

a. enlarged cisterna magna
b. normal cisterna magna
c. normal cerebellum
d. enlarged cerebellum

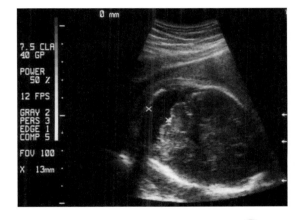

Obstetrics / Second and Third Trimesters

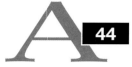

A. Enlarged cisterna magna.

The cisterna magna is a fluid-filled space between the cerebellum and posterior cranium. The cisterna magna should not measure more than 10 mm. The cisterna magna depicted in this image measures 13 mm, which is considered enlarged.

▶ Baun J: *Ob/Gyn Sonography: An Illustrated Review*. Pasadena, CA, Davies Publishing, 2016, p 118.
▶ Gill KA: *Ultrasound in Obstetrics and Gynecology: A Practitioner's Guide*. Pasadena, CA, Davies Publishing, 2014, p 126.

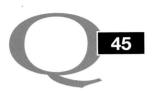

In this image the arrow points to:

a. third ventricle
b. fourth ventricle
c. choroid plexus
d. cavum septi pellucidi

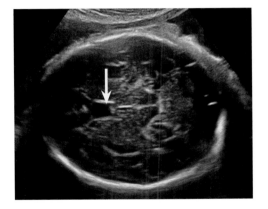

Obstetrics / Second and Third Trimesters / AIT—Hotspot

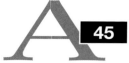

D. Cavum septi pellucidi.

▶ Baun J: *Ob/Gyn Sonography: An Illustrated Review*. Pasadena, CA, Davies Publishing, 2016, p 114.

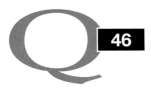

In this image the arrow points to:

a. cavum septi pellucidi
b. choroid plexus
c. cerebral peduncles
d. thalamus

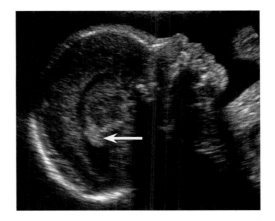

Obstetrics / Second and Third Trimesters / AIT—Hotspot

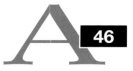

B. Choroid plexus.

This sagittal image demonstrates a normal fetal head at the level of the lateral ventricle. Although this particular view is not typically obtained as part of a routine second/third trimester protocol, it is important to know the normal structures. The arrow is pointing to the choroid plexus in the atrium of the lateral ventricle.

▶ Baun J: *Ob/Gyn Sonography: An Illustrated Review*. Pasadena, CA, Davies Publishing, 2016, p 115.

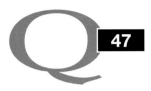 **47**

The site where the body, posterior, and temporal horns of the lateral ventricle converge is called the:

a. pons
b. third ventricle
c. choroid
d. atrium

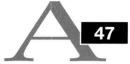

D. Atrium.

In the brain, the *atrium* (plural, *atria*) of the lateral ventricle is where the body, posterior, and temporal horns of the lateral ventricle meet. It is the site of the bulk of the choroid plexus in the lateral ventricle.

▶ Baun J: *Ob/Gyn Sonography: An Illustrated Review*. Pasadena, CA, Davies Publishing, 2016, p 115.

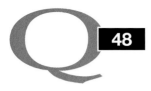

In this image the arrow points to:

a. cerebellar hemispheres
b. cerebral peduncles
c. cerebral hemispheres
d. cisterna magna

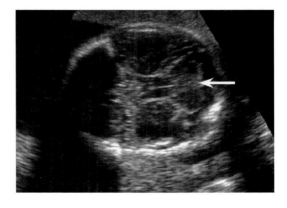

Obstetrics / Second and Third Trimesters / AIT—Hotspot

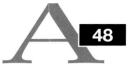

A. Cerebellar hemispheres.

The cerebellum (consisting of the cerebellar hemispheres) is located in the posterior cranial fossa. It lies posteroinferiorly in the skull, anterior to the fluid-filled cisterna magna.

▶ Baun J: *Ob/Gyn Sonography: An Illustrated Review*. Pasadena, CA, Davies Publishing, 2016, p 114.

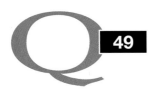

49

The development of the corpus callosum is normally complete by weeks:

a. 21–25
b. 26–30
c. 31–36
d. 16–20

Obstetrics / Second and Third Trimesters

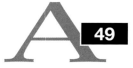

D. 16–20.

The corpus callosum should be fully developed by the end of week 17, although authors vary, with some saying it can take up to 22 weeks. Although the corpus callosum is usually not well documented by prenatal sonography, its absence can be associated with colpocephaly (enlarged, tear-shaped lateral ventricles) and enlarged occipital horns as well as Dandy-Walker syndrome, in which a posterior fossa cyst is identified.

- Baun J: *Ob/Gyn Sonography: An Illustrated Review*. Pasadena, CA, Davies Publishing, 2016, p 114.
- Callen PW: *Ultrasonography in Obstetrics and Gynecology*, 5th edition. Philadelphia, Elsevier, 2008, p 355.
- Sliman MH, Gill KA: The first trimester. In Gill KA: *Ultrasound in Obstetrics and Gynecology: A Practitioner's Guide*. Pasadena, CA, Davies Publishing, 2014, p 235.

50

The portion of dura mater that invaginates along the intercerebral fissure is called the:

a. cavum septi pellucidi
b. third ventricle
c. aqueduct of Sylvius
d. falx cerebri

Obstetrics / Second and Third Trimesters

A **50**

D. Falx cerebri.

The *falx cerebri* (or simply *falx*) is formed by an invagination of the dura mater. The falx separates the left cerebral hemisphere from the right. It is absent in the presence of pathologies such as alobar holoprosencephaly, hydranencephaly, and anencephaly.

▶ Baun J: *Ob/Gyn Sonography: An Illustrated Review*. Pasadena, CA, Davies Publishing, 2016, p 117.

51

The anastomotic network of arteries located at the base of the brain is the:

a. circle of Willis
b. Sylvian fissure
c. posterior cerebral artery
d. vertebrobasilar circulation

Obstetrics / Second and Third Trimesters

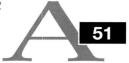

A. Circle of Willis.

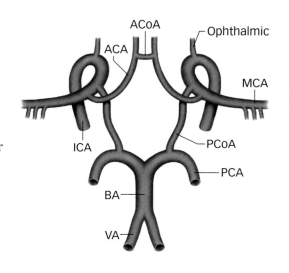

The circle of Willis, located at the base of the brain anterior to the brainstem, is shaped like a traffic circle of blood vessels. In the presence of an obstruction, it serves as a safety mechanism for blood flow through the fetal (and, later, adult) brain. The circle is formed by the anterior communicating artery (ACoA), anterior cerebral arteries (ACA), posterior communicating arteries (PCoA), and posterior cerebral arteries (PCA). Also depicted are the basilar artery (BA), vertebral arteries (VA), internal carotid arteries (ICA), and middle cerebral arteries (MCA).

▶ Baun J: *Ob/Gyn Sonography: An Illustrated Review*. Pasadena, CA, Davies Publishing, 2016, p 118.

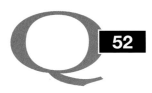

What is the name of the symmetric midline intracranial structure whose lateral walls are formed by the inferior aspect of the thalamus and hypothalamus?

a. corpus callosum
b. third ventricle
c. fourth ventricle
d. aqueduct of Sylvius

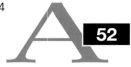

B. Third ventricle.

The third ventricle lies in the midline, inferior to the lateral ventricles. It is connected to the lateral ventricles via the foramen of Monro. The third ventricle commonly lies between the two lobes of the thalamus.

▶ Baun J: *Ob/Gyn Sonography: An Illustrated Review*. Pasadena, CA, Davies Publishing, 2016, pp 115–116.

The fluid-filled structure located between the cerebellum and the occipital bone in the posterior fossa is the:

a. cisterna magna
b. third ventricle
c. fourth ventricle
d. interpeduncular cistern

A 53

A. Cisterna magna.

The cisterna magna is a fluid-filled space in the posterior fossa behind the cerebellum. The maximal anterior–posterior size is 10 mm. Measurements greater than 10 mm should be considered suspicious for Dandy-Walker malformation or another pathologic process.

Baun J: *Ob/Gyn Sonography: An Illustrated Review*. Pasadena, CA, Davies Publishing, 2016, pp 117–118.

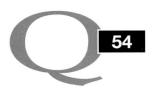# 54

In the fetus, how many ossification centers does each vertebra develop?

a. 5
b. 4
c. 3
d. 2

Obstetrics / Second and Third Trimesters

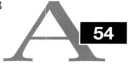

C. 3.

The three ossification centers are the centrum, or vertebral body, and two laminae laterally.

- Baun J: *Ob/Gyn Sonography: An Illustrated Review*. Pasadena, CA, Davies Publishing, 2016, p 119.
- Gill KA: *Ultrasound in Obstetrics and Gynecology: A Practitioner's Guide*. Pasadena, CA, Davies Publishing, 2014, p 123.

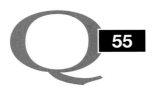
55

Approximately when do the ossification centers of the fetal spine become sonographically visible?

a. 10 weeks
b. 18 weeks
c. 22 weeks
d. 16 weeks

Obstetrics / Second and Third Trimesters

A 55

D. 16 weeks.

By 16 weeks all three ossification centers of the fetal spine are visible by sonography.

▶ Baun J: *Ob/Gyn Sonography: An Illustrated Review*. Pasadena, CA, Davies Publishing, 2016, p 119.
▶ Gill KA: *Ultrasound in Obstetrics and Gynecology: A Practitioner's Guide*. Pasadena, CA, Davies Publishing, 2014, p 123.

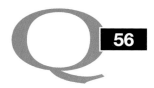

In this image what structure is identified by the arrow?

a. pulmonary artery
b. pulmonary vein
c. aortic root
d. inferior vena cava

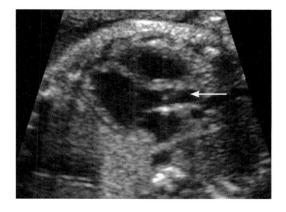

Obstetrics / Second and Third Trimesters / AIT—Hotspot

A **56**

C. Aortic root.

This view is the left ventricular outflow tract (LVOT) view, which features the left atrium, mitral valve, left ventricle, and aorta with its aortic valve. The arrow is pointing to the aortic root.

▶ Baun J: *Ob/Gyn Sonography: An Illustrated Review*. Pasadena, CA, Davies Publishing, 2016, p 161.

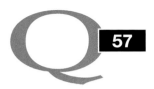

In this image what structure is identified by the arrow?

a. left atrium
b. right atrium
c. pulmonary artery
d. superior vena cava

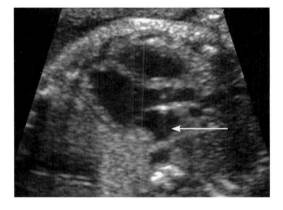

Obstetrics / Second and Third Trimesters / AIT—Hotspot

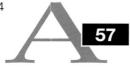

A. Left atrium.

This image is a left ventricular outflow tract (LVOT) view, which features the left atrium, mitral valve, left ventricle, and aorta with its aortic valve. The arrow is pointing to the left atrium.

▶ Baun J: *Ob/Gyn Sonography: An Illustrated Review*. Pasadena, CA, Davies Publishing, 2016, p 163.

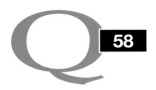

In this image of a normal four-chamber heart, the cardiac structure closest to the fetal spine is the:

a. left ventricle
b. right atrium
c. left atrium
d. right ventricle

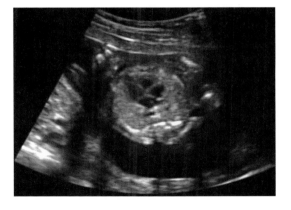

Obstetrics / Second and Third Trimesters / AIT—Hotspot

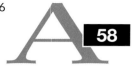

C. Left atrium.

The left atrium is always the chamber closest to the spine in a normal four-chamber view of the fetal heart.

- Baun J: *Ob/Gyn Sonography: An Illustrated Review*. Pasadena, CA, Davies Publishing, 2016, p 162.
- Gill KA: Fetal syndromes. In Gill KA: *Ultrasound in Obstetrics and Gynecology: A Practitioner's Guide*. Pasadena, CA, Davies Publishing, 2014, p 127.

Q 59

This image of the fetal heart depicts the:

a. ductus arteriosus
b. aortic arch
c. right ventricular outflow tract
d. inferior vena cava

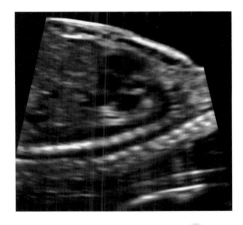

Obstetrics / Second and Third Trimesters / AIT—Hotspot

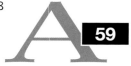

B. Aortic arch.

Note the "candy cane" appearance and the small head and neck branches. The aortic arch is easiest to visualize in the sagittal plane, when the fetus is spine-up; however, a good view can also be obtained in this plane when the fetus is spine-down.

▶ Baun J: *Ob/Gyn Sonography: An Illustrated Review*. Pasadena, CA, Davies Publishing, 2016, p 161.
▶ Rodriguez J, Gill KA: The second and third trimesters: basic and targeted scans. In Gill KA: *Ultrasound in Obstetrics and Gynecology: A Practitioner's Guide*. Pasadena, CA, Davies Publishing, 2014, p 156.

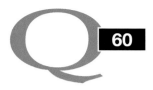

When imaging the fetal heart, what valve do you see between the left atrium and left ventricle?

a. aortic
b. mitral
c. pulmonary
d. tricuspid

Obstetrics / Second and Third Trimesters

A **60**

B. Mitral.

The mitral valve is a bicuspid atrioventricular valve located between the left atrium and the left ventricle.

▶ Baun J: *Ob/Gyn Sonography: An Illustrated Review*. Pasadena, CA, Davies Publishing, 2016, p 162.

▶ Rodriguez J, Gill KA: The second and third trimesters: basic and targeted scans. In Gill KA: *Ultrasound in Obstetrics and Gynecology: A Practitioner's Guide*. Pasadena, CA, Davies Publishing, 2014, pp 127–128, 150, 152, 153, 159.

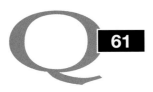

121

Q 61

The right ventricle, pulmonary semilunar valve, pulmonary artery, and right atrium are demonstrated in the:

a. four-chamber view of the heart
b. five-chamber view of the heart
c. right ventricular outflow tract view
d. left ventricular outflow tract view

Obstetrics / Second and Third Trimesters

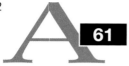

C. Right ventricular outflow tract view.

The right ventricular outflow tract (RVOT) view demonstrates the right atrium, right ventricle, pulmonary valve, main pulmonary artery, and ductus arteriosus. The aorta is also visualized in cross section.

- Baun J: *Ob/Gyn Sonography: An Illustrated Review*. Pasadena, CA, Davies Publishing, 2016, p 164.
- Rodriguez J, Gill KA: The second and third trimesters: basic and targeted scans. In Gill KA: *Ultrasound in Obstetrics and Gynecology: A Practitioner's Guide*. Pasadena, CA, Davies Publishing, 2014, pp 151, 155.

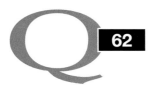

The arrow in this image is pointing to what structure?

a. ductus arteriosus
b. aorta
c. right pulmonary artery
d. inferior vena cava

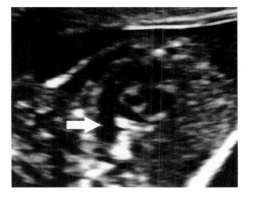

Obstetrics / Second and Third Trimesters / AIT—Hotspot

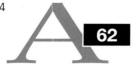

A. Ductus arteriosus.

This image is the right ventricular outflow tract (RVOT) view. The main pulmonary artery branches into the left and right pulmonary arteries and ductus arteriosus. The RVOT view demonstrates the right pulmonary artery and ductus arteriosus.

▶ Rodriguez J, Gill KA: The second and third trimesters: basic and targeted scans. In Gill KA: *Ultrasound in Obstetrics and Gynecology: A Practitioner's Guide*. Pasadena, CA, Davies Publishing, 2014, pp 155–156.

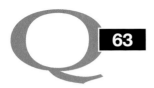

Which view of the fetal heart is demonstrated here?

a. aortic arch
b. right atrial inflow
c. left ventricular outflow tract
d. ductal arch

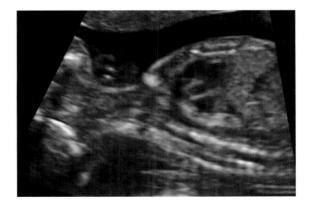

Obstetrics / Second and Third Trimesters

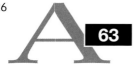

D. Ductal arch.

This image, known as a *ductal arch view*, is a long-axis view of the ductus arteriosus entering the descending aorta. The flat shape of the ductal arch and the origin of the main pulmonary artery from the anteriorly located right heart indicate which view this is.

▶ Baun J: *Ob/Gyn Sonography: An Illustrated Review*. Pasadena, CA, Davies Publishing, 2016, p 518.
▶ Gill KA: The second and third trimesters: basic and targeted scans. In Gill KA: *Ultrasound in Obstetrics and Gynecology: A Practitioner's Guide*. Pasadena, CA, Davies Publishing, 2014, p 156.

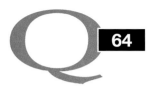

What pathology is demonstrated in this image of the fetal chest at the level of the heart in this fetus with trisomy 18?

a. pericardial effusion
b. diaphragmatic hernia
c. pleural effusion
d. cardiac anomaly

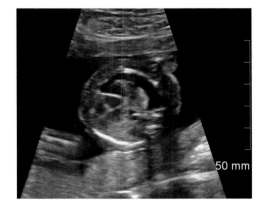

Obstetrics / Second and Third Trimesters

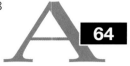

C. Pleural effusion.

This four-chamber view of the fetal heart demonstrates a pleural effusion in a hydropic fetus with trisomy 18 (Edwards syndrome). In addition to the pleural effusion, note the skin thickening around the thorax. There may be a cardiac anomaly in this fetus, but it is not demonstrated in this image.

▶ Baun J: *Ob/Gyn Sonography: An Illustrated Review*. Pasadena, CA, Davies Publishing, 2016, pp 166–167.
▶ Gill KA: Anomalies associated with polyhydramnios. In Gill KA: *Ultrasound in Obstetrics and Gynecology: A Practitioner's Guide*. Pasadena, CA, Davies Publishing, 2014, pp 244–245.

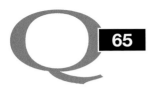

What is the most common type of congenital diaphragmatic hernia?

a. right-sided hernia
b. bilateral hernias
c. both sides with equal frequency
d. left-sided hernia

Obstetrics / Second and Third Trimesters

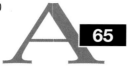

D. Left-sided hernia.

Left-sided congenital diaphragmatic hernia (CDH) is five times more common than right-sided CDH. Nevertheless, the right diaphragm and hemithorax should always be examined as part of an anatomic scan.

- Baun J: *Ob/Gyn Sonography: An Illustrated Review*. Pasadena, CA, Davies Publishing, 2016, p 168.
- Raatz Stephenson S (ed): *Diagnostic Medical Sonography: Obstetrics and Gynecology*, 3rd edition. Baltimore, Lippincott Williams & Wilkins, 2012, ch 21.

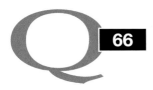

Which of the following is the proper term for the chief finding in this image?

a. dextrocardia
b. levocardia
c. dextroposition
d. levoposition

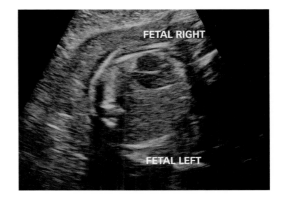

Obstetrics / Second and Third Trimesters

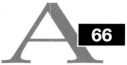

C. Dextroposition.

In this fetus with a large left-sided diaphragmatic hernia, the heart has been displaced to the right. This is termed *dextroposition*. *Levoposition* means that the heart is located in the left side of the chest. There is also *mesocardia* demonstrated in the image because the apex is pointed neither left nor right. *Dextrocardia* means that the apex of the heart is pointed toward the right. *Levocardia* means that the apex of the heart is pointed to the left.

▶ Baun J: *Ob/Gyn Sonography: An Illustrated Review*. Pasadena, CA, Davies Publishing, 2016, pp 168–169.
▶ Gill KA: Anomalies associated with polyhydramnios. In Gill KA: *Ultrasound in Obstetrics and Gynecology: A Practitioner's Guide*. Pasadena, CA, Davies Publishing, 2014, p 162.
▶ Otto CM: Textbook of clinical echocardiography, 5th edition. Philadelphia, Elsevier Saunders, 2013, pp 448–449.

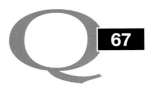

In this image the arrow points to:

a. hepatic vein
b. ductus venosus
c. umbilical vein
d. right portal vein

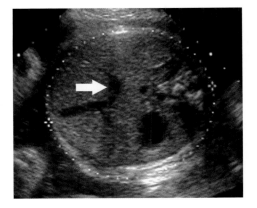

Obstetrics / Second and Third Trimesters / AIT—Hotspot

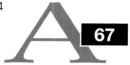

D. Right portal vein.

The "hockey stick" landmark is formed by the confluence of the umbilical vein and left and right portal veins. The inferior vena cava is seen in cross section in this view, adjacent to the aorta.

- Baun J: *Ob/Gyn Sonography: An Illustrated Review*. Pasadena, CA, Davies Publishing, 2016, p 222.
- Mavrides E, Moscoso G, Carvalho JS, et al: The anatomy of the umbilical, portal and hepatic venous systems in the human fetus at 14–19 weeks of gestation. Ultrasound Obstet Gynecol 18:598–604, 2001.

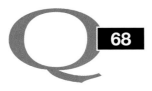

Q 68

Fetal bowel echogenicity is:

a. more echogenic than bone and less echogenic than liver
b. less echogenic than bone and more echogenic than liver
c. more echogenic than liver and less echogenic than spleen
d. more echogenic than spleen and isoechoic with liver

Obstetrics / Second and Third Trimesters

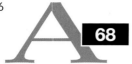

B. Less echogenic than bone and more echogenic than liver.

Normal fetal bowel may be heterogeneous, but its overall brightness should not be echogenic compared to the fetal bone.

▶ Baun J: *Ob/Gyn Sonography: An Illustrated Review*. Pasadena, CA, Davies Publishing, 2016, pp 225, 235.

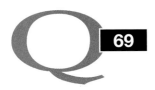

The anatomic relationships demonstrated in this image document the presence and integrity of the:

a. spleen
b. liver
c. diaphragm
d. gallbladder

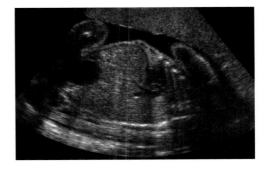

Obstetrics / Second and Third Trimesters

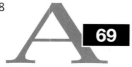

C. Diaphragm.

The diaphragm can be visualized as a hypoechoic linear structure in the sagittal view of the fetal chest and abdomen.

- Baun J: *Ob/Gyn Sonography: An Illustrated Review*. Pasadena, CA, Davies Publishing, 2016, p 160.
- Magner RG Jr, Vance CA: Ultrasound of the normal fetal chest. abdomen, and pelvis. In Raatz Stephenson S (ed): *Diagnostic Medical Sonography: Obstetrics and Gynecology*, 3rd edition. Philadelphia, Lippincott Williams & Wilkins, 2012, ch 20.

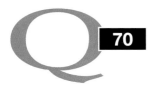

In this image the arrow points to:

a. stomach
b. gallbladder
c. renal cyst
d. ovarian cyst

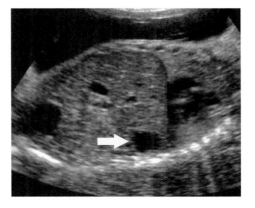

Obstetrics / Second and Third Trimesters / AIT—Hotspot

A 70

A. Stomach.

This anechoic circular structure immediately inferior to the diaphragm represents a normal fetal stomach.

▶ Baun J: *Ob/Gyn Sonography: An Illustrated Review*. Pasadena, CA, Davies Publishing, 2016, p 224.

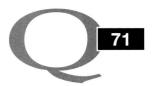

In this black-and-white rendering of a color Doppler image obtained at the level of the abdominal cord insertion, blood flow is demonstrated in which vessels?

a. hepatic veins

b. umbilical veins

c. ductus venosus

d. umbilical arteries

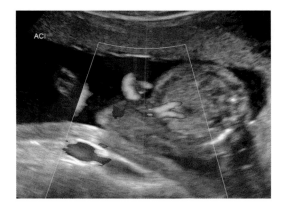

Obstetrics / Second and Third Trimesters / AIT—Hotspot

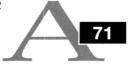

D. Umbilical arteries.

This color Doppler image (rendered here in black and white) was taken at the level of the abdominal cord insertion, where the two umbilical arteries enter the fetal pelvis and join the iliac arteries.

▶ Baun J: *Ob/Gyn Sonography: An Illustrated Review*. Pasadena, CA, Davies Publishing, 2016, p 223.

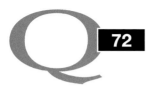

Q 72

Which of the following statements about the ulna is TRUE when you are observing the fetal forearm in the anatomic position?

a. The ulna is positioned lateral to the radius.
b. The ulna is on the same side as the thumb.
c. The ulna is longer than the radius proximally.
d. The ulna is shorter and thicker than the radius.

Obstetrics / Second and Third Trimesters

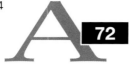

C. The ulna is longer than the radius proximally.

- Baun J: *Ob/Gyn Sonography: An Illustrated Review*. Pasadena, CA, Davies Publishing, 2016, p 199.
- Rodriguez J, Gill KA: The second and third trimesters: basic and targeted scans. In Gill KA: *Ultrasound in Obstetrics and Gynecology: A Practitioner's Guide*. Pasadena, CA, Davies Publishing, 2014, p 165.

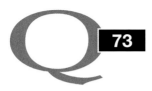

145

Ossification of fetal long bones begins at the:

a. epiphyses
b. metaphysis
c. centrum
d. middle of the shaft at the diaphysis

Obstetrics / Second and Third Trimesters

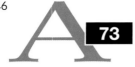

D. Middle of the shaft at the diaphysis.

Fetal ossification of the long bones begins with the diaphysis—the long, thin part of the bone.

▶ Baun J: *Ob/Gyn Sonography: An Illustrated Review*. Pasadena, CA, Davies Publishing, 2016, p 79.
▶ Gill KA: Anomalies associated with polyhydramnios. In Gill KA: *Ultrasound in Obstetrics and Gynecology: A Practitioner's Guide*. Pasadena, CA, Davies Publishing, 2014, p 260.

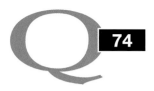

This image best demonstrates:

a. normal ossified epiphysis
b. femoral bowing
c. micromelia
d. normal ossified metaphysis

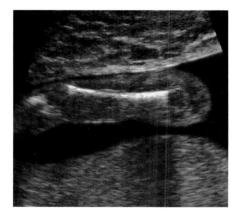

Obstetrics / Second and Third Trimesters

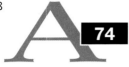

D. Normal ossified metaphysis.

The *metaphysis*, or growth plate, is the portion of the bone between the *epiphysis* (the junction of the calcified shaft with the cartilaginous end of the bone) and the thin part of the *diaphysis* (the shaft).

▶ Baun J: *Ob/Gyn Sonography: An Illustrated Review*. Pasadena, CA, Davies Publishing, 2016, p 209.

Q 75

A fetus with the feet presenting is in which fetal position?

a. complete breech
b. footling breech
c. cephalic
d. frank breech

Obstetrics / Second and Third Trimesters

A **75**

B. Footling breech.

Complete breech is the term used when the fetal buttocks are presenting and the legs are crossed. *Frank* or *rump breech* occurs when the buttocks are presenting and the fetal legs are flexed with feet near the fetal face. *Cephalic* is the opposite of breech, referring to the head as the presenting part.

▶ Baun J: *Ob/Gyn Sonography: An Illustrated Review*. Pasadena, CA, Davies Publishing, 2016, p 331.

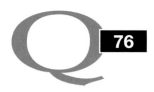

Of the following, which is NOT a type of fetal lie?

a. transverse
b. longitudinal
c. cephalic
d. oblique

Obstetrics / Second and Third Trimesters

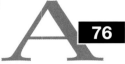

C. Cephalic.

Fetal position is determined by both fetal lie and fetal presentation. *Fetal lie* describes the relationship of the longitudinal axis of the fetus to the longitudinal axis of the mother and can be any of the listed choices EXCEPT cephalic. *Fetal presentation* describes the part of the fetus that is expected to be delivered first, and there are many variations, including cephalic, breech, shoulder, and others.

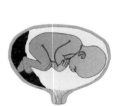
Transverse lie

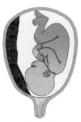
Cephalic presentation

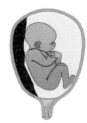
Complete breech presentation

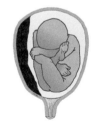
Frank breech presentation

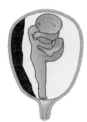
Footling breech presentation

▶ Baun J: *Ob/Gyn Sonography: An Illustrated Review*. Pasadena, CA, Davies Publishing, 2016, pp 330–331.

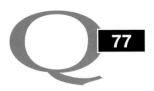

Which fetal biophysical profile score indicates that all sonographic parameters are normal?

a. 6
b. 10
c. 12
d. 8

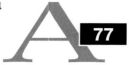

D. 8.

A biophysical profile using the Manning scoring system is based on a 10-point scale. Two of the points are for the nonstress test, which is not a sonographic parameter. The other 8 points are determined by ultrasound. A passing sore includes 2 points for fetal breathing, 2 points for fetal movement, 2 points for fetal tone, and 2 points for amniotic fluid. A score of zero is assigned if the fetus does not perform a specific parameter in the required fashion.

▶ Baun J: *Ob/Gyn Sonography: An Illustrated Review*. Pasadena, CA, Davies Publishing, 2016, p 83.

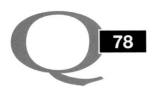

Q 78

In a normal fetal biophysical profile, the single deepest pocket of amniotic fluid should measure:

a. >2 cm
b. >4 cm
c. >6 cm
d. >8 cm

Obstetrics / Second and Third Trimesters

A 78

A. >2 cm.

In order to earn 2 points for amniotic fluid, there must be at least one vertical pocket of fluid measuring at least 2 cm. (Other terms for the single deepest pocket are *maximum vertical pocket* and *deepest vertical pocket*.)

▶ Baun J: *Ob/Gyn Sonography: An Illustrated Review*. Pasadena, CA, Davies Publishing, 2016, p 83.

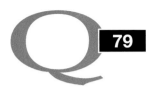

The criterion for a reactive (normal) nonstress test (NST) is:

a. one 15-second FHR (fetal heart rate) acceleration lasting at least 15 seconds over 15 minutes
b. one 15-second FHR acceleration lasting at least 15 seconds over 30 minutes
c. two 15-second FHR accelerations lasting at least 15 seconds over 40 minutes
d. two 15-second FHR accelerations lasting at least 15 seconds over 20 minutes

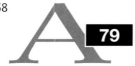

D. Two 15-second FHR accelerations lasting at least 15 seconds over 20 minutes.

The NST involves monitoring both fetal heart rate and uterine contractions using a dedicated nonstress test machine. Fetal heart rate should have beat-to-beat variability and demonstrate two accelerations of more than 15 bpm lasting at least 15 seconds over a 20-minute period.

- Baun J: *Ob/Gyn Sonography: An Illustrated Review*. Pasadena, CA, Davies Publishing, 2016, p 83.
- Callen PW: *Ultrasonography in Obstetrics and Gynecology*, 5th edition. Philadelphia, Elsevier, 2008, p 782.

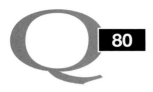

This image depicts:

a. female genitalia
b. anomalous genitalia
c. ambiguous genitalia
d. male genitalia

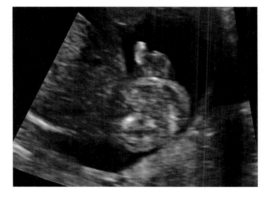

Obstetrics / Second and Third Trimesters

D. Male genitalia.

The scrotum and penis are visualized in this image of a 19-week fetus. The testicles do not appear because they do not descend into the scrotum until about 28 weeks' gestation.

▶ Baun J: *Ob/Gyn Sonography: An Illustrated Review*. Pasadena, CA, Davies Publishing, 2016, p 250.

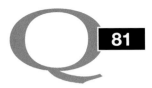

This view of the fetal face demonstrates the:

a. nostrils
b. mouth
c. lenses
d. mandible

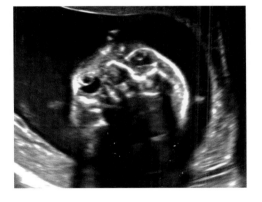

Obstetrics / Second and Third Trimesters

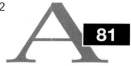

C. Lenses.

Visualizing the lenses demonstrates that eyes are present in the orbits.

- Baun J: *Ob/Gyn Sonography: An Illustrated Review*. Pasadena, CA, Davies Publishing, 2016, pp 90, 96–99.
- Rodriguez J, Gill KA: The second and third trimesters: basic and targeted scans. In Gill KA: *Ultrasound in Obstetrics and Gynecology: A Practitioner's Guide*. Pasadena, CA, Davies Publishing, 2014, pp 147–148.

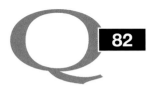

This three-dimensional surface rendering depicts what fetal anomaly?

a. unilateral cleft lip
b. hypotelorism
c. micrognathia
d. cebocephaly

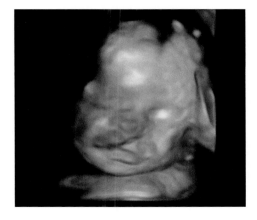

Obstetrics / Second and Third Trimesters

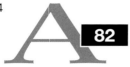

A. Unilateral cleft lip.

This 3D ultrasound image shows a fetus with a unilateral cleft lip. The palate is not visualized in this surface-rendered view. *Hypotelorism* refers to closely spaced orbits, *micrognathia* to a small chin, and *cebocephaly* to a single central nostril.

- Baun J: *Ob/Gyn Sonography: An Illustrated Review*. Pasadena, CA, Davies Publishing, 2016, pp 92–95.
- Rodriguez J, Gill KA: The second and third trimesters: basic and targeted scans. In Gill KA: *Ultrasound in Obstetrics and Gynecology: A Practitioner's Guide*. Pasadena, CA, Davies Publishing, 2014, pp 144–145.

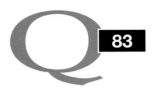 83

A targeted scan is ordered to evaluate a pregnancy for:

a. gender
b. anomalies
c. multiple gestation
d. placental location

Obstetrics / Second and Third Trimesters

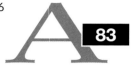

B. Anomalies.

A targeted scan will be ordered to enhance detection of abnormalities in a high-risk pregnancy. The indications for a targeted scan include (among many others) substance abuse, maternal compromise because of infection or conditions such as diabetes, and advanced maternal age.

- Baun J: *Ob/Gyn Sonography: An Illustrated Review*. Pasadena, CA, Davies Publishing, 2016, pp 92–95.
- Rodriguez J, Gill KA: The second and third trimesters: basic and targeted scans. In Gill KA: *Ultrasound in Obstetrics and Gynecology: A Practitioner's Guide*. Pasadena, CA, Davies Publishing, 2014, pp 120, 140–168.

Targeted scans are usually overseen by which physician specialist?

a. radiologist
b. obstetrician
c. perinatologist
d. pathologist

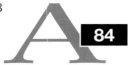

C. Perinatologist.

A perinatologist is an obstetrician who specializes in high-risk pregnancies or patients at risk for having a high-risk pregnancy. These physicians undergo a fellowship in perinatology after completing their residency in obstetrics and gynecology.

▶ Rodriguez J, Gill KA: The second and third trimesters: basic and targeted scans. In Gill KA: *Ultrasound in Obstetrics and Gynecology: A Practitioner's Guide*. Pasadena, CA, Davies Publishing, 2014, p 141.

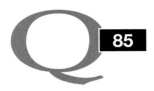
Q 85

The fetal component of the placenta develops from the:

a. decidua basalis
b. chorionic villi
c. decidua vera
d. amnion

Obstetrics / Placenta

A 85

B. Chorionic villi.

The *villous chorion* (or *chorionic villi*) forms the fetal part of the placenta.

▶ Baun J: *Ob/Gyn Sonography: An Illustrated Review*. Pasadena, CA, Davies Publishing, 2016, pp 33–34.

▶ Baun J, Gill KA: The placenta and umbilical cord. In Gill KA: *Ultrasound in Obstetrics and Gynecology: A Practitioner's Guide*. Pasadena, CA, Davies Publishing, 2014, p 180.

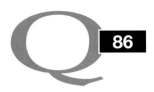

The normal anteroposterior (AP) thickness of a full-term placenta should NOT exceed:

a. 4 cm
b. 3 cm
c. 5 cm
d. 6 cm

Obstetrics / Placenta

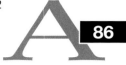

A. 4 cm.

Placental thickness should not exceed 4 cm in AP diameter. A thickened placenta may result from fetal conditions such as hydrops or maternal conditions such as diabetes.

▶ Baun J: *Ob/Gyn Sonography: An Illustrated Review*. Pasadena, CA, Davies Publishing, 2016, pp 35, 36.

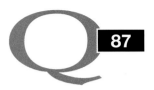

87

The placental edge should be at least how far from the internal cervical os to indicate that the mother is NOT at increased risk for complications during delivery.

a. 1.0 cm

b. 2.0 cm

c. 1.5 cm

d. 2.5 cm

Obstetrics / Placenta

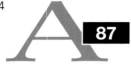

B. 2.0 cm.

The placental edge should be at least 2.0 cm (20 mm) from the internal os of the cervix to confirm that the mother is at least risk for bleeding during delivery.

▶ Baun J: *Ob/Gyn Sonography: An Illustrated Review*. Pasadena, CA, Davies Publishing, 2016, p 42.
▶ Baun J, Gill KA: The placenta and umbilical cord. In Gill KA: *Ultrasound in Obstetrics and Gynecology: A Practitioner's Guide*. Pasadena, CA, Davies Publishing, 2014, pp 194–196.

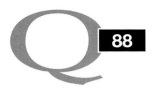

In this transverse image of an asymptomatic pregnant uterus, which would best describe the placental location?

a. posterior
b. anterior
c. fundal
d. lateral

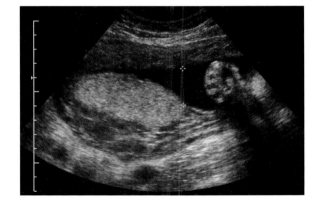

Obstetrics / Placenta

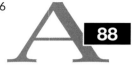

A. Posterior.

Location of the placenta can be described as anterior, posterior, lateral, or fundal. In some cases both a longitudinal and a transverse image are needed to determine the location more accurately. In this image, though, the placenta is clearly in a posterior position.

▶ Baun J, Gill KA: The placenta and umbilical cord. In Gill KA: *Ultrasound in Obstetrics and Gynecology: A Practitioner's Guide*. Pasadena, CA, Davies Publishing, 2014, p 188.

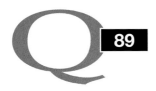

Decidua refers to the:

a. myometrium
b. endometrium
c. perimetrium
d. uterine cavity

Obstetrics / Placenta

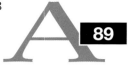

B. Endometrium.

The *decidua* is the term used for the functional layer of the endometrium after conception occurs. *Myometrium* is the muscle layer of the uterus. *Perimetrium* is the thin, serosal outer layer.

▶ Baun J, Gill KA: The placenta and umbilical cord. In Gill KA: *Ultrasound in Obstetrics and Gynecology: A Practitioner's Guide*. Pasadena, CA, Davies Publishing, 2014, p 179.

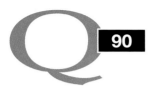

90

What is the term for an accessory lobe of the placenta that is located apart from the main placental body?

a. succenturiate
b. circumvallate
c. circummarginate
d. annular

Obstetrics / Placenta

A 90

A. Succenturiate.

A succenturiate lobe of the placenta is a piece of placenta connected to the main part of the placenta by a membrane. It is important to document a succenturiate placenta because its presence increases the risk of vasa previa or retained placenta during delivery.

Baun J: *Ob/Gyn Sonography: An Illustrated Review*. Pasadena, CA, Davies Publishing, 2016, p 39.

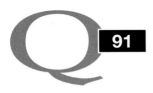

Q 91

The maternal surface of the placenta is called the:

a. decidua vera
b. decidua basalis
c. decidua parietalis
d. decidua capsularis

Obstetrics / Placenta

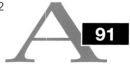

B. Decidua basalis.

During early pregnancy, the *decidua capsularis* is the part of the endometrium covering the blastocyst. *Decidua vera* and *decidua parietalis* are alternative terms for the endometrium covering the cavity.

▶ Baun J: *Ob/Gyn Sonography: An Illustrated Review*. Pasadena, CA, Davies Publishing, 2016, p 7.
▶ Sliman MH, Gill KA: The first trimester. In Gill KA: *Ultrasound in Obstetrics and Gynecology: A Practitioner's Guide*. Pasadena, CA, Davies Publishing, 2014, p 92.

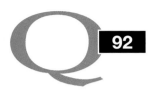

A placenta that has two equally sized lobes connected by vessels is called a:

a. circumvallate placenta
b. bipartite placenta
c. membranous placenta
d. lobar placenta

Obstetrics / Placenta

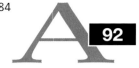

B. Bipartite placenta.

A bipartite placenta is very similar to a placenta with a succenturiate lobe except that with a bipartite placenta the two lobes are roughly equal in size. The umbilical cord connects into the main lobe. As with a succenturiate lobe, it is important to rule out vasa previa with transvaginal ultrasound when bipartite placentation is suspected.

▶ Baun J: *Ob/Gyn Sonography: An Illustrated Review*. Pasadena, CA, Davies Publishing, 2016, pp 39–40.
▶ Baun J, Gill KA: The placenta and umbilical cord. In Gill KA: *Ultrasound in Obstetrics and Gynecology: A Practitioner's Guide*. Pasadena, CA, Davies Publishing, 2014, p 193.

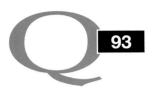

The amnion and chorion usually fuse by weeks:

a. 8–11
b. 10–14
c. 12–16
d. 14–18

Obstetrics / Placenta

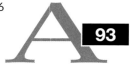

C. 12–16.

Fusion of the amnion and chorion in some cases may be delayed until 16 weeks, but these membranes should not be seen separately after that. They usually fuse by 12 weeks.

▶ Sliman MH, Gill KA: The first trimester. In Gill KA: *Ultrasound in Obstetrics and Gynecology: A Practitioner's Guide*. Pasadena, CA, Davies Publishing, 2014, p 93.

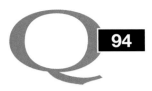

Q 94

Amnionicity refers to the number of:

a. placentas
b. outer sacs
c. inner sacs
d. fetuses

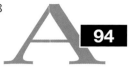

C. Inner sacs.

Amnionicity refers to the number of inner sacs. *Chorionicity* refers to number of placentas or outer sacs, and *zygosity* refers to the number of eggs fertilized.

- Baun J: *Ob/Gyn Sonography: An Illustrated Review*. Pasadena, CA, Davies Publishing, 2016, p 312.
- Gill KA: Multiple gestations and their complications. In Gill KA: *Ultrasound in Obstetrics and Gynecology: A Practitioner's Guide*. Pasadena, CA, Davies Publishing, 2014, p 293.

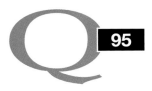

Ultrasonography of an 18-week fetus demonstrates that the fetus is missing a hand. What is the most likely diagnosis?

a. failure of amnion-chorion fusion
b. amniotic band sequence
c. limb–body wall complex
d. Arnold-Chiari malformation

Obstetrics / Placenta

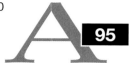

B. Amniotic band sequence.

In the absence of other fetal malformations, amniotic band sequence (or syndrome) is the most likely cause of a solitary missing extremity or any of its parts. The culprit is a free-floating piece of amnion. With limb–body wall complex there are severe malformations and a very disrupted fetus. An Arnold-Chiari malformation relates to myelomeningocele. Failure of the chorion and amnion to fuse does not cause limb abnormalities.

- Baun J: *Ob/Gyn Sonography: An Illustrated Review*. Pasadena, CA, Davies Publishing, 2016, pp 287–288.
- Baun J, Gill KA: The placenta and umbilical cord. In Gill KA: *Ultrasound in Obstetrics and Gynecology: A Practitioner's Guide*. Pasadena, CA, Davies Publishing, 2014, pp 182–183.

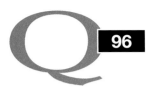

96

What is the name for a placenta in which a loose chorionic membrane folds back upon itself and encircles the fetal surface?

a. circumvallate
b. circummarginate
c. succenturiate
d. annular

Obstetrics / Placenta

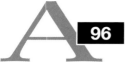

A. Circumvallate.

A circumvallate placenta is one whose edge folds back upon itself, leaving some of the placenta extrachorial. This type of placentation places the pregnancy at increased risk for premature rupture of membranes, growth restriction, and abruption.

▶ Baun J: *Ob/Gyn Sonography: An Illustrated Review*. Pasadena, CA, Davies Publishing, 2016, p 38.

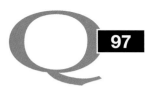

Q 97

What is the most common vascular abnormality of the umbilical cord?

a. four-vessel cord
b. cord cyst
c. short cord
d. single umbilical artery (SUA)

Obstetrics / Placenta

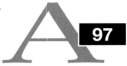

D. Single umbilical artery (SUA).

When there is only a single umbilical artery (SUA) instead of the normal two, the fetus is said to have a two-vessel cord (2VC). The normal umbilical cord has two arteries and one vein. Although SUA can be an incidental finding, it may also be associated with abnormal chromosomes and congenital anomalies.

▶ Baun J: *Ob/Gyn Sonography: An Illustrated Review*. Pasadena, CA, Davies Publishing, 2016, p 57.

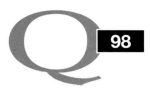

98

Using color Doppler imaging you confirm the presence of umbilical cord between the internal cervical os and the fetal presenting part. What is this condition?

a. vasa previa
b. battledore placenta
c. nuchal cord
d. velamentous insertion

Obstetrics / Placenta

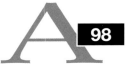

A. Vasa previa.

Vasa previa is a clinically serious condition, since it places a patient going into active labor at risk for a tear in the large umbilical vessel and certain catastrophic hemorrhaging if surgical intervention is not initiated immediately. Vasa previa can be the result of a *velamentous insertion* (a cord that attaches beyond the placental edge and into the free membranes of the placenta) or an abnormality of vessels that extend from the placenta. In a *battledore placenta*, the cord inserts along the margin of the placenta. The term *nuchal cord* refers to the umbilical cord wrapped around the fetal neck.

▶ Allen LM: Abnormalities of the placenta and umbilical cord. In Raatz Stephenson S (ed): *Diagnostic Medical Sonography: Obstetrics and Gynecology*, 3rd edition. Philadelphia, Lippincott Williams & Wilkins, 2012, ch 18.
▶ Baun J: *Ob/Gyn Sonography: An Illustrated Review*. Pasadena, CA, Davies Publishing, 2016, p 45.

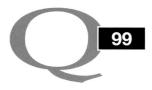

Q 99

The umbilical cord consists of:

a. one artery and two veins
b. two arteries and one vein
c. one artery and one vein
d. two arteries and two veins

Obstetrics / Placenta

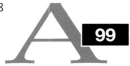

B. Two arteries and one vein.

> The normal umbilical cord has two umbilical arteries and one umbilical vein. This is termed a *three-vessel cord* (3VC).

▶ Baun J: *Ob/Gyn Sonography: An Illustrated Review*. Pasadena, CA, Davies Publishing, 2016, p 54.

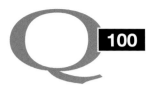

100

What is the function of the umbilical vein?

a. to carry deoxygenated blood from the placenta to the fetus
b. to carry oxygenated blood from the placenta to the fetus
c. to carry oxygenated blood from the fetus to the placenta
d. to carry deoxygenated blood from the fetus to the placenta

Obstetrics / Placenta

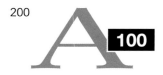

B. To carry oxygenated blood from the placenta to the fetus.

The umbilical vein connects the placenta to the fetus. Maternal oxygenated blood is sent to the fetus via the umbilical vein. Once it enters the fetus, this oxygenated blood bypasses the liver via the ductus venosus and is sent to the right heart.

▶ Baun J: *Ob/Gyn Sonography: An Illustrated Review*. Pasadena, CA, Davies Publishing, 2016, p 54.

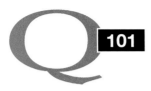

201

101

Which of the following are the two most common clinical manifestations of trophotropism?

a. battledore placenta and velamentous insertion
b. battledore placenta and two-vessel cord
c. battledore placenta and single umbilical vein
d. battledore placenta and single umbilical artery

Obstetrics / Placenta

A 101

A. Battledore placenta and velamentous insertion.

Trophotropism describes the process of how the placenta prefers areas of the myometrium with the greatest blood supply. Placenta that is adherent to areas of poor blood supply tends to atrophy. Therefore, rather than being inserted centrally, the cord may appear to be marginal or velamentous.

▶ Baun J: *Ob/Gyn Sonography: An Illustrated Review*. Pasadena, CA, Davies Publishing, 2016, p 60.

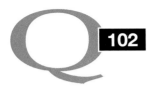

What does this power Doppler image demonstrate?

a. normal cord
b. nuchal cord
c. cord entanglement
d. tethered cord

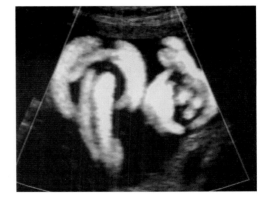

Obstetrics / Placenta

A 102

C. Cord entanglement.

Cord entanglement is possible in a monoamniotic (i.e., monochorionic/monoamniotic) twin pregnancy, in which both fetuses are in the same amniotic sac. Cord entanglement can result in cord compression and fetal demise. Nuchal cord occurs when the umbilical cord becomes coiled around the fetal neck.

▶ Baun J: *Ob/Gyn Sonography: An Illustrated Review*. Pasadena, CA, Davies Publishing, 2016, p 60.

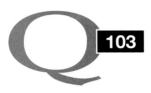

Which fetal vessel(s) in the fetal pelvis help identify the umbilical cord?

a. umbilical arteries
b. umbilical vein
c. hepatic vein
d. iliac arteries

Obstetrics / Placenta

A 103

D. Iliac arteries.

The normal umbilical cord is made up of two umbilical arteries and a single umbilical vein. The umbilical arteries originate from the iliac arteries and course alongside the fetal bladder to enter the umbilical cord. There should be one umbilical artery on either side of the fetal bladder.

▶ Baun J: *Ob/Gyn Sonography: An Illustrated Review*. Pasadena, CA, Davies Publishing, 2016, p 55.
▶ Callen PW: *Ultrasonography in Obstetrics and Gynecology*, 5th edition. Philadelphia, Elsevier, 2008, pp 745–746.

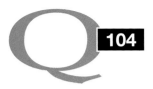

This image was obtained in a healthy, asymptomatic patient at 28 weeks' gestation and represents:

a. cystic hygroma
b. placental teratoma
c. umbilical cord cysts
d. uterine synechiae

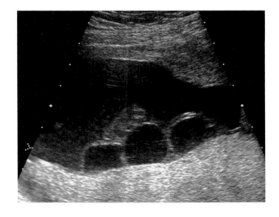

Obstetrics / Placenta

A **104**

C. Umbilical cord cysts.

True cysts of the umbilical cord are common and do not usually cause any problems with the fetus. These cysts, which usually resolve on their own, may be from dilatation of either the allantoic duct or the vitelline/omphalomesenteric duct.

▶ Baun J: *Ob/Gyn Sonography: An Illustrated Review*. Pasadena, CA, Davies Publishing, 2016, pp 62–63.

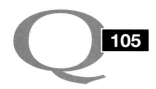

What type of placental cord insertion (PCI) is demonstrated in this image?

a. marginal
b. velamentous
c. membranous
d. central

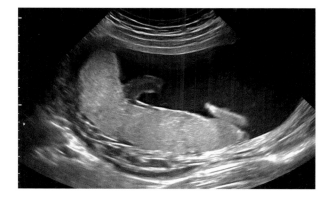

Obstetrics / Placenta

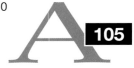

D. Central.

This image is a classic example of a typical central placental cord insertion (PCI). Marginal cord insertions occur when the PCI is near the edge of the placenta. Velamentous and membranous cord insertions are dangerous because the umbilical cord does not insert into the placenta and there is a risk of vasa previa.

- Baun J: *Ob/Gyn Sonography: An Illustrated Review*. Pasadena, CA, Davies Publishing, 2016, p 60.
- Baun J, Gill KA: The placenta and umbilical cord. In Gill KA: *Ultrasound in Obstetrics and Gynecology: A Practitioner's Guide*. Pasadena, CA, Davies Publishing, 2014, pp 202, 206–207.

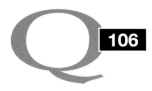

211

This image is from a 30-year-old pregnant patient who was a victim of physical domestic violence. She reported to the emergency room with cramping in her lower abdomen. Based on the clinical history and image provided, what diagnosis is most likely?

a. retroplacental abruption
b. placental villous lake
c. placental infarct
d. placenta accreta

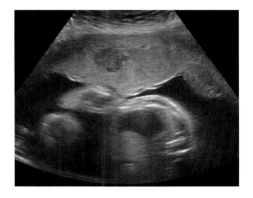

Obstetrics / Placenta / AIT—PACSim

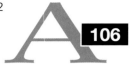

A. Retroplacental abruption.

Given a history of trauma and a hypoechoic mass near the maternal surface of the placenta, abruption (*abruptio placentae*) should be considered.

- Baun J: *Ob/Gyn Sonography: An Illustrated Review*. Pasadena, CA, Davies Publishing, 2016, p 45.
- Baun J, Gill KA: The placenta and umbilical cord. In Gill KA: *Ultrasound in Obstetrics and Gynecology: A Practitioner's Guide*. Pasadena, CA, Davies Publishing, 2014, pp 196–197.

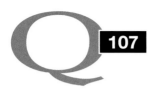

107

Premature separation of the placenta from the myometrium is called:

a. placenta previa
b. placental abruption
c. placenta percreta
d. placenta accreta

Obstetrics / Placenta

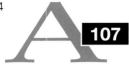

B. Placental abruption.

Placental abruption occurs when part of the placenta detaches from the maternal myometrium. It may be associated with bleeding if the abruption is toward the edge of the placenta, or occult if the hemorrhage is retroplacental. Placental abruption is potentially fatal to the fetus and can be difficult to diagnose by ultrasound, especially if retroplacental.

▶ Baun J: *Ob/Gyn Sonography: An Illustrated Review*. Pasadena, CA, Davies Publishing, 2016, pp 45–46.

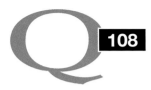

108

What is the term for a clinically serious condition in which velamentously inserted cord vessels precede the fetal presenting part?

a. complete previa
b. vasa previa
c. partial previa
d. prolapsed cord

Obstetrics / Placenta

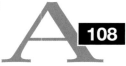

B. Vasa previa.

Vasa previa is a potentially lethal condition in which membranes containing fetal vessels traverse the internal os of the cervix. Vasa previa may occur with succenturiate lobe and velamentous cord insertion, and it must be ruled out when either of these conditions is present. *Prolapsed cord* occurs when the umbilical cord precedes the fetus as the presenting part. Although prolapse is also a potentially serious complication, it is separate from vasa previa. *Complete* or *partial previa* occurs when the placenta encroaches upon the internal os of the cervix.

▶ Baun J: *Ob/Gyn Sonography: An Illustrated Review*. Pasadena, CA, Davies Publishing, 2016, p 45.

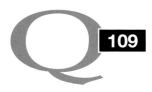

A patient presents with a recent history of bright red vaginal bleeding, and transabdominal sonography yields this image. The most likely diagnosis is:

a. placenta percreta
b. partial placenta previa
c. placental abruption
d. complete placenta previa

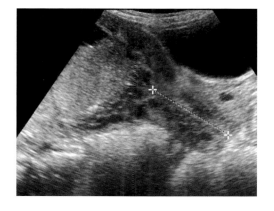

Obstetrics / Placenta / AIT—PACSim

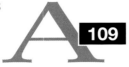

D. Complete placenta previa.

Previa usually presents as painless vaginal bleeding. This image is suggestive of complete placenta previa because the placental body crosses the internal os of the cervix. However, in this image there is partial bladder filling, which may cause an error in documenting the true location of the placental edge. Transvaginal ultrasound must be performed to image the internal os in order to check for placenta previa.

▶ Baun J: *Ob/Gyn Sonography: An Illustrated Review*. Pasadena, CA, Davies Publishing, 2016, pp 42–43.

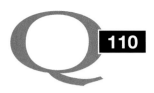

219

A vascular tumor of the chorion is referred to as:

a. angioma
b. hemangioma
c. chorioangioma
d. angiomyoma

Obstetrics / Placenta

A 110

C. Chorioangioma.

A *chorioangioma* is a benign, nontrophoblastic vascular tumor originating from the chorion. Chorioangiomas vary in size but usually are located on the fetal surface of the placenta. Large (>5 cm) *hemangiomas* may cause fetal hydrops because of their increased vascularity and are also associated with polyhydramnios, preterm labor, and intrauterine growth restriction.

▶ Baun J: *Ob/Gyn Sonography: An Illustrated Review*. Pasadena, CA, Davies Publishing, 2016, p 49.

▶ Baun J, Gill KA: The placenta and umbilical cord. In Gill KA: *Ultrasound in Obstetrics and Gynecology: A Practitioner's Guide*. Pasadena, CA, Davies Publishing, 2014, pp 199–200.

▶ Callen PW: *Ultrasonography in Obstetrics and Gynecology*, 5th edition. Philadelphia, Elsevier, 2008, pp 742–745.

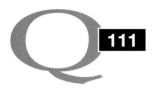

221

A patient presented with spotting at 24 weeks' gestation. Transvaginal ultrasound was performed to confirm the placental location. What are the findings in this ultrasound image?

a. fundal placenta
b. placenta covering internal os
c. placenta 0–20 mm from internal os
d. placenta >20 mm from internal os

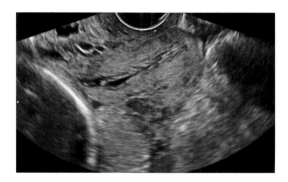

Obstetrics / Placenta

A 111

C. Placenta 0–20 mm from internal os.

This image presents a placenta that is encroaching on the internal os of the cervix, consistent with placenta previa. Although the placenta is not completely covering the internal os, it is about 10 mm from the internal os, which may necessitate a cesarean section to reduce the risk of hemorrhage.

▶ Baun J: *Ob/Gyn Sonography: An Illustrated Review*. Pasadena, CA, Davies Publishing, 2016, pp 42–45.

▶ Baun J, Gill KA: The placenta and umbilical cord. In Gill KA: *Ultrasound in Obstetrics and Gynecology: A Practitioner's Guide*. Pasadena, CA, Davies Publishing, 2014, p 194.

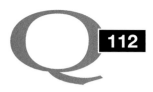

112

When is placental infarction a cause of concern?

a. when the infarction is peripheral in location
b. when it cannot be imaged
c. when it covers more than 30% of the placenta
d. when it is accompanied by subchorionic cysts

Obstetrics / Placenta

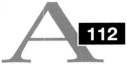

C. When it covers more than 30% of the placenta.

Placental infarctions result from ischemic necrosis of placental villi caused by interference with maternal blood flow to the intervillous space. Often part of the normal placental aging process, they are usually peripherally located and rarely are a cause of concern if uteroplacental circulation is otherwise normal. In severe cases placental insufficiency may develop, accompanied by massive blood and fibrin deposition that extends into the intervillous space. Blood collections covering 30%–40% of the placenta may result in fetal growth restriction or even demise. Placental infarctions are not usually visible on sonograms, although they may sometimes appear as echogenic; however, they cannot be sonographically differentiated from retroplacental hematoma.

- Baun J: *Ob/Gyn Sonography: An Illustrated Review*. Pasadena, CA, Davies Publishing, 2016, pp 41–42.
- Baun J, Gill KA: The placenta and umbilical cord. In Gill KA: *Ultrasound in Obstetrics and Gynecology: A Practitioner's Guide*. Pasadena, CA, Davies Publishing, 2014, pp 190–191.

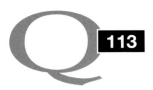

How would you grade this placenta with a few scattered bright echoes, slight indentations at the chorionic plate, and an unchanged basal layer?

a. grade 0
b. grade I
c. grade II
d. grade III

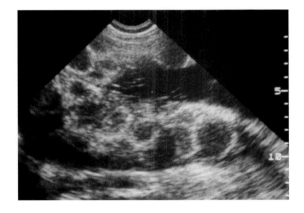

Obstetrics / Placenta

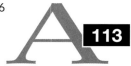

D. Grade III.

As shown in this image, Grannum's grade III placenta displays large calcifications and indentations of the basal plate.

- Baun J: *Ob/Gyn Sonography: An Illustrated Review*. Pasadena, CA, Davies Publishing, 2016, p 37.
- Baun J, Gill KA: The placenta and umbilical cord. In Gill KA: *Ultrasound in Obstetrics and Gynecology: A Practitioner's Guide*. Pasadena, CA, Davies Publishing, 2014, pp 188–190.

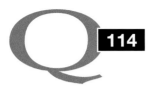

The diastolic notch is best described as:

a. early diastolic flow reduction
b. flow reversal in early diastole
c. flow reversal in late diastole
d. late diastolic flow reduction

Obstetrics / Placenta

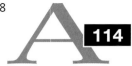

A. Early diastolic flow reduction.

The diastolic notch—distinct from the dicrotic notch referenced in peripheral vascular Doppler studies—is a brief deflection of a spectral waveform obtained from the uterine artery during early diastole. While the hemodynamic mechanism for creation of a diastolic notch is unclear, its appearance early in gestation suggests compromise of placental circulation.

▶ Baun J, Gill KA: The placenta and umbilical cord. In Gill KA: *Ultrasound in Obstetrics and Gynecology: A Practitioner's Guide*. Pasadena, CA, Davies Publishing, 2014, p 376.

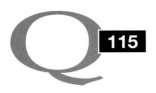
115

In performing a uterine artery Doppler study, you should place the spectral range gate (sample volume):

a. near its origin at the internal iliac artery
b. mid-vessel, with strongest color signal
c. near the cervix
d. anywhere along its course

Obstetrics / Placenta

A **115**

C. Near the cervix.

All of the protocols employing uterine artery Doppler as an indicator of gestational integrity obtain spectral waveforms from a site near the cervix. Samples should be obtained from uterine arteries on both sides.

▶ Baun J: *Ob/Gyn Sonography: An Illustrated Review*. Pasadena, CA, Davies Publishing, 2016, pp 358–359.
▶ Gill KA: *Ultrasound in Obstetrics and Gynecology: A Practitioner's Guide*. Pasadena, CA, Davies Publishing, 2014, pp 385–387.

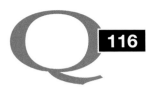

Fetal–maternal metabolic exchange in the placenta occurs at the level of the:

a. decidua
b. cotyledons
c. lobes
d. villi

Obstetrics / Placenta

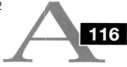

D. Villi.

The villi are the functioning parts of the placenta that exchange oxygen and nutrients with the spiral arteries of the maternal circulation.

▶ Baun J: *Ob/Gyn Sonography: An Illustrated Review*. Pasadena, CA, Davies Publishing, 2016, p 33.

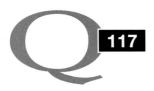

Q 117

Which of the following forms the placenta?

a. chorion laeve
b. oocyte
c. decidua capsularis
d. chorion frondosum

Obstetrics / Placenta

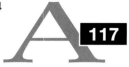

D. Chorion frondosum.

The *decidua basalis* becomes the maternal portion of the placenta; the *chorion frondosum*, also known as the *villous chorion*, is the fetal part of the placenta. The *chorion laeve* constitutes the smooth chorion, just deep to the *decidua capsularis*, which is the layer that covers the blastocyst after implantation. The *oocyte*—the immature ovum or egg cell—is the female gamete.

▶ Baun J: *Ob/Gyn Sonography: An Illustrated Review*. Pasadena, CA, Davies Publishing, 2016, p 32.
▶ Baun J, Gill KA: The placenta and umbilical cord. In Gill KA: *Ultrasound in Obstetrics and Gynecology: A Practitioner's Guide*. Pasadena, CA, Davies Publishing, 2014, p 180.

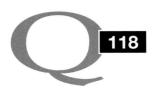

The placenta takes over progesterone production from what structure/organ?

a. chorion frondosum
b. corpus luteum
c. oocyte
d. fallopian tube

Obstetrics / Placenta

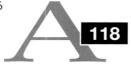

B. Corpus luteum.

The corpus luteum cyst of pregnancy secretes progesterone in order to sustain the developing pregnancy. As the placenta forms and produces progesterone, the corpus luteum involutes and regresses, usually by 12–16 weeks (although some authors allow up to 18–20 weeks for the corpus luteum cyst of pregnancy to resolve completely).

- Baun J: *Ob/Gyn Sonography: An Illustrated Review*. Pasadena, CA, Davies Publishing, 2016, p 386.
- Gill KA: *Ultrasound in Obstetrics and Gynecology: A Practitioner's Guide*. Pasadena, CA, Davies Publishing, 2014, pp 33, 101.
- Morgan MA, Jones J: Corpus luteum. Radiopaedia. Available at http://radiopaedia.org/articles/corpus-luteum.

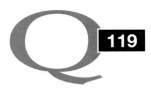

The condition characterized by the deep invasion of placental villi into the myometrium but not the serosal layer is called:

a. placenta percreta
b. chorioangioma
c. placenta increta
d. placental abruption

Obstetrics / Placenta

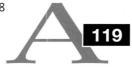

C. Placenta increta.

Placenta increta is one of three types of morbidly adherent placenta. With increta, the placenta invades the myometrium but does not penetrate the serosal layer of the uterus. *Placenta accreta* is less invasive than placenta increta. *Placental abruption* is a tearing away of the placenta from the uterus, and *chorioangioma* is a placental tumor.

- Abuhamad A: Morbidly adherent placenta. Semin Perinatol 37:359–364, 2013.
- Baun J: *Ob/Gyn Sonography: An Illustrated Review*. Pasadena, CA, Davies Publishing, 2016, pp 47–49.

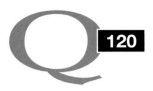

Which term describes a condition of the placenta in which the villi penetrate through the serosal layer of the uterus, possibly with bladder invasion?

a. percreta
b. circumvallate
c. battledore
d. annular

Obstetrics / Placenta

A 120

A. Percreta.

Placenta percreta is a condition in which the placenta penetrates the serosal layer of the myometrium, with placental vessels on the surface of the uterus. These placental vessels can invade the bladder and may be visualized with cystoscopy. *Battledore placenta* is another name for a placenta with a marginal cord insertion. An *annular placenta* is one that attaches only at the periphery, and a *circumvallate placenta* is one in which the outer edge is rolled up.

▶ Baun J: *Ob/Gyn Sonography: An Illustrated Review*. Pasadena, CA, Davies Publishing, 2016, p 47.

▶ Shipp TD: Sonographic evaluation of the placenta. In Rumack CM (ed): *Diagnostic Ultrasound*, 4th edition. St. Louis, Mosby, 2011, pp 1499–1526.

The earliest measure of sonographically demonstrable gestational age is:

a. biparietal diameter
b. mean sac diameter
c. yolk sac size
d. crown-rump length

Obstetrics / Assessment of Gestational Age

A 121

B. Mean sac diameter.

The first sign of intrauterine pregnancy is a gestational sac. The mean sac diameter (MSD), which is the average of three orthogonal measurements of the sac, gives the approximate gestational age.

▶ Baun J: *Ob/Gyn Sonography: An Illustrated Review*. Pasadena, CA, Davies Publishing, 2016, pp 69–70.

Using an endovaginal approach, the sonographer can identify a gestational sac within the uterine cavity as early as:

a. 3.5 menstrual weeks
b. 4.5 menstrual weeks
c. 5.0 menstrual weeks
d. 5.5 menstrual weeks

Obstetrics / Assessment of Gestational Age

A 122

B. 4.5 menstrual weeks.

With endovaginal ultrasound the earliest an intrauterine sac can be visualized is at 4.5 menstrual weeks. At this gestational age a yolk sac will not yet be seen. Until the yolk sac is visualized, at 5.0–5.5 weeks, an intrauterine pregnancy cannot be confirmed.

▶ Baun J: *Ob/Gyn Sonography: An Illustrated Review*. Pasadena, CA, Davies Publishing, 2016, pp 8, 9, 12.

What is the most accurate measurement of gestational age during the first trimester?

a. crown-rump length
b. biparietal diameter
c. mean sac diameter
d. yolk sac size

Obstetrics / Assessment of Gestational Age

A 123

A. Crown-rump length.

Up to 10 weeks' menstrual age, the CRL is accurate to within a few days and therefore is the most accurate means of dating a pregnancy. Although mean sac diameter is used very early in the pregnancy, once CRL can be measured it is a more accurate measure of age than any other means during the first trimester. After 10 weeks' gestational age, the biparietal diameter (BPD), head circumference (HC), abdominal circumference (AC), and femur length (FL) are used to date the pregnancy.

▶ Baun J: *Ob/Gyn Sonography: An Illustrated Review*. Pasadena, CA, Davies Publishing, 2016, p 68.

124

Which plane of section through the fetal head is used to obtain a biparietal diameter measurement?

a. sagittal
b. occipital
c. cephalic
d. transaxial

Obstetrics / Assessment of Gestational Age

A 124

D. Transaxial.

The *transaxial plane*, also known as the *transverse* or *axial plane*, is a true cross section of the fetal head. *Biparietal* means from one parietal bone to the other. In order to obtain a biparietal diameter (BPD), a transaxial plane must be used.

▶ Baun J: *Ob/Gyn Sonography: An Illustrated Review*. Pasadena, CA, Davies Publishing, 2016, p 72.

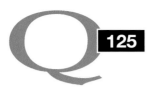
125

The cerebellum is visualized during an attempt to measure the BPD. In which direction, in relation to the fetus, does the transducer need to be moved in order to obtain a proper BPD?

a. caudad
b. lateral
c. medial
d. cephalad

Obstetrics / Assessment of Gestational Age

A 125

D. Cephalad.

The transducer needs to be moved in a more cephalad direction, toward the top of the fetal head. The cerebellum is at the most inferior point of the fetal skull, in the occipital part of the cerebrum.

▶ Baun J: *Ob/Gyn Sonography: An Illustrated Review*. Pasadena, CA, Davies Publishing, 2016, pp 72–73.

▶ Rodriguez J, Gill KA: The second and third trimesters: basic and targeted scans. In Gill KA: *Ultrasound in Obstetrics and Gynecology: A Practitioner's Guide*. Pasadena, CA, Davies Publishing, 2014, p 125.

When obtaining a femur length measurement, what should you include in the measurement?

a. diaphysis
b. femoral head
c. condyles
d. epiphysis

Obstetrics / Assessment of Gestational Age

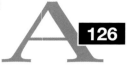

A. Diaphysis.

The *diaphysis* is the shaft of the femur and is the part of the bone that is measured as part of the femur length. The femoral head and epiphyses should not be included in the measurement.

- Baun J: *Ob/Gyn Sonography: An Illustrated Review*. Pasadena, CA, Davies Publishing, 2016, pp 76–79.
- Rodriguez J, Gill KA: The second and third trimesters: basic and targeted scans. In Gill KA: *Ultrasound in Obstetrics and Gynecology: A Practitioner's Guide*. Pasadena, CA, Davies Publishing, 2014, pp 136–137.

A gain setting that is too high can cause what problem when you are measuring femur length?

a. increased shadowing from bone
b. overestimation of femur length
c. increased exposure to ultrasound energy
d. increased heat production in bone

Obstetrics / Assessment of Gestational Age

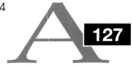

B. Overestimation of femur length.

Technical settings are a crucial part of performing ultrasound examinations. Proper settings of the gain, focal zones, and other technical factors all contribute to an optimal image.

▶ Baun J: *Ob/Gyn Sonography: An Illustrated Review*. Pasadena, CA, Davies Publishing, 2016, pp 76–79.
▶ Hagen-Ansert SL (ed): *Textbook of Diagnostic Ultrasonography*, 7th edition. St. Louis, Elsevier Mosby, 2012, pp 1151–1152.

Abdominal circumference measurements are most useful in assessing:

a. normal somatic growth of the fetus
b. gestational age
c. estimated date of confinement (EDC)
d. fetal oxygenation

Obstetrics / Assessment of Gestational Age

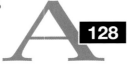

A. Normal somatic growth of the fetus.

The abdominal circumference (AC) helps measure how well the fetal body is growing. Somatic growth is used with other biometric parameters to determine EDC and gestational age. Although the AC alone does not provide direct information on fetal oxygenation, the HC/AC ratio can provide information that may be lead to suspicions of intrauterine growth restriction, which may be the result of a hypoxia situation, among other causes.

▶ Baun J: *Ob/Gyn Sonography: An Illustrated Review*. Pasadena, CA, Davies Publishing, 2016, pp 75–76.

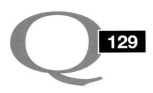

257

When you measure the abdominal circumference (AC), which of the following should appear in the image?

a. heart
b. stomach
c. kidneys
d. umbilical cord insertion

Obstetrics / Assessment of Gestational Age

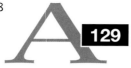

B. Stomach.

The AC measurement should include the stomach and the portal vein. The kidneys, heart, and umbilical cord insertion site should not be included in the AC image.

- Baun J: *Ob/Gyn Sonography: An Illustrated Review*. Pasadena, CA, Davies Publishing, 2016, pp 75–76.
- Rodriguez J, Gill KA: The second and third trimesters: basic and targeted scans. In Gill KA: *Ultrasound in Obstetrics and Gynecology: A Practitioner's Guide*. Pasadena, CA, Davies Publishing, 2014, p 129.

259

How does maternal diabetes affect fetal abdominal circumference (AC)?

a. Diabetes makes the amount of fetal body fat increase, causing an enlarged AC.
b. Diabetes makes the stomach dilate, causing an enlarged AC.
c. Diabetes makes the AC smaller than normal due to malnutrition.
d. Diabetes makes the intestines swell, causing an enlarged AC.

Obstetrics / Assessment of Gestational Age

A 130

A. Diabetes makes the amount of fetal body fat increase, causing an enlarged AC.

Maternal diabetes may cause *macrosomia*, an increased fetal weight. The AC is elevated in patients with maternal diabetes because although glucose will go through the placenta, the insulin does not, and therefore the fetus experiences hyperglycemia.

▶ Baun J: *Ob/Gyn Sonography: An Illustrated Review*. Pasadena, CA, Davies Publishing, 2016, pp 322–324.

▶ Gill KA: Maternal disorders and pregnancy. In Gill KA: *Ultrasound in Obstetrics and Gynecology: A Practitioner's Guide*. Pasadena, CA, Davies Publishing, 2014, pp 319–328.

131

Which of the following landmarks should be visualized in the proper axial plane required for both biparietal diameter (BPD) and head circumference (HC)?

a. cerebellum
b. Sylvian fissure
c. cavum septi pellucidi
d. orbits

Obstetrics / Assessment of Gestational Age

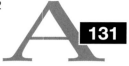

C. Cavum septi pellucidi.

The proper axial plane required for measurement of BPD or HC should include the cavum septi pellucidi, falx cerebri, and thalamic nuclei. The fetal orbits and cerebellum should not be in the plane.

▶ Baun J: *Ob/Gyn Sonography: An Illustrated Review*. Pasadena, CA, Davies Publishing, 2016, pp 72, 73.

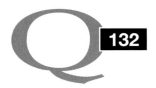

In this fetus with severe oligohydramnios, the head has adopted a shape that corresponds to a cephalic index of 64%. What is the name of this shape?

a. brachycephaly
b. cloverleaf skull
c. dolichocephaly
d. strawberry skull

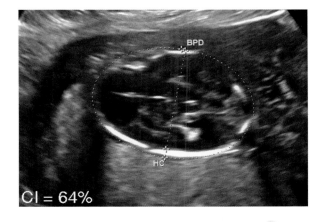

Obstetrics / Assessment of Gestational Age

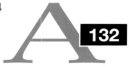

C. Dolichocephaly.

A dolichocephalic skull shape is long and narrow. The normal cephalic index (CI)—the ratio of the biparietal diameter to the occipitofrontal diameter, or BPD/OFD (multiplied by 100 to yield a percentage)—is between 74% and 83%. A cephalic index less than 74% indicates dolichocephaly; in this case the fetus has a CI of 64% and is dolichocephalic. Dolichocephaly may occur as a result of severe oligohydramnios, which can cause compression of the skull.

▶ Baun J: *Ob/Gyn Sonography: An Illustrated Review*. Pasadena, CA, Davies Publishing, 2016, p 75.
▶ Gill KA: *Ultrasound in Obstetrics and Gynecology: A Practitioner's Guide*. Pasadena, CA, Davies Publishing, 2014, pp 135, 286, 307, 352.

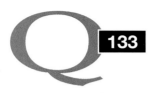
133

The fetal transcerebellar diameter in millimeters is equivalent to fetal menstrual age in weeks at approximately what menstrual age?

a. 12–16 weeks
b. 14–20 weeks
c. 18–22 weeks
d. 20–24 weeks

Obstetrics / Assessment of Gestational Age

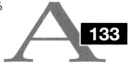

B. 14–20 weeks.

The transcerebellar diameter in millimeters is roughly equivalent to the menstrual age between approximately 14 and 20 weeks. Abnormal measurement of the cerebellum may be seen with some chromosomal anomalies and cerebellar defects.

- Baun J: *Ob/Gyn Sonography: An Illustrated Review*. Pasadena, CA, Davies Publishing, 2016, p 81.
- Rodriguez J, Gill KA: The second and third trimesters: basic and targeted scans. In Gill KA: *Ultrasound in Obstetrics and Gynecology: A Practitioner's Guide*. Pasadena, CA, Davies Publishing, 2014, p 127.

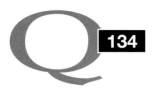

An increase in intraorbital distance above the 95th percentile indicates which facial anomaly?

a. anophthalmia
b. hypotelorism
c. hypertelorism
d. cyclopia

Obstetrics / Assessment of Gestational Age

A 134

C. Hypertelorism.

A condition in which fetal eyes are too far apart (greater than the 95th percentile) is termed *hypertelorism*. Although hypertelorism can be a normal variant, it is also associated with congenital anomalies such as encephalocele and median cleft anomalies.

▶ Baun J: *Ob/Gyn Sonography: An Illustrated Review*. Pasadena, CA, Davies Publishing, 2016, p 96.

What is the proper method for measuring fetal binocular distance?

a. the width of one orbit
b. from outer margin to outer margin of the orbits
c. the distance between the orbits
d. from outer lens to outer lens

Obstetrics / Assessment of Gestational Age

A 135

B. From outer margin to outer margin of the orbits.

The *binocular distance* (BD), also known as the *outer orbital distance* (OOD), is measured from the outer margin of one orbit to the outer margin of the contralateral orbit. The distance between the inner margins of the orbits is called the *inner orbital* (also *interorbital* or *interocular*) *diameter* (IOD).

▶ Baun J: *Ob/Gyn Sonography: An Illustrated Review*. Pasadena, CA, Davies Publishing, 2016, pp 96–99.
▶ Gill KA: *Ultrasound in Obstetrics and Gynecology: A Practitioner's Guide*. Pasadena, CA, Davies Publishing, 2014, pp 147, 340.

Q 136

The cephalic index is performed to identify:

a. growth restriction
b. gestational age
c. brain volume
d. head shape

Obstetrics / Assessment of Gestational Age

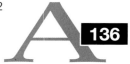

D. Head shape.

The cephalic index (CI) is a calculation performed to determine if the head shape is normal. Abnormal head shapes include brachycephaly and dolichocephaly.

- Baun J: *Ob/Gyn Sonography: An Illustrated Review*. Pasadena, CA, Davies Publishing, 2016, p 75.
- Rodriguez J, Gill KA: The second and third trimesters: basic and targeted scans. In Gill KA: *Ultrasound in Obstetrics and Gynecology: A Practitioner's Guide*. Pasadena, CA, Davies Publishing, 2014, p 135.

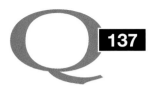

Which measurement is better than biparietal diameter when you are estimating menstrual age in a dolichocephalic fetus?

a. biparietal diameter
b. head circumference
c. BPD/AC ratio
d. cephalic index

Obstetrics / Assessment of Gestational Age

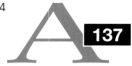

B. Head circumference.

A dolichocephalic head will yield biparietal diameter values lower than those appropriate for gestational age, while a brachycephalic head will produce values that are greater than expected. The *cephalic index* (CI) is a useful measure of the reliability of standard biparietal diameter: If the cephalic index varies by more than one standard deviation (SD) above or below the expected value, then the head circumference is a more reliable indicator of gestational age than is the biparietal diameter. (See also the answer to question 138.)

▶ Baun J: *Ob/Gyn Sonography: An Illustrated Review*. Pasadena, CA, Davies Publishing, 2016, p 75.

Q 138

Which of the following is used to calculate the cephalic index (CI)?

a. BPD/AC × 100
b. (BPD + OFD) × 0.523
c. BPD/OFD × 100
d. BPD/HC

Obstetrics / Assessment of Gestational Age

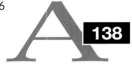

C. BPD/OFD × 100.

> The calculation for CI is BPD/OFD × 100, which yields a percentage. The CI is automatically calculated in most OB packages, but it is important to know the equation. The CI should be documented whenever an unusual head shape, such as dolichocephaly or brachycephaly, is suspected. A CI less than 74% indicates dolichocephaly; a CI greater than 83% indicates brachycephaly.

▶ Baun J: *Ob/Gyn Sonography: An Illustrated Review*. Pasadena, CA, Davies Publishing, 2016, p 75.
▶ Rodriguez J, Gill KA: The second and third trimesters: basic and targeted scans. In Gill KA: *Ultrasound in Obstetrics and Gynecology: A Practitioner's Guide*. Pasadena, CA, Davies Publishing, 2014, p 135.

139

A normal nuchal fold thickness measurement is:

a. <6 mm
b. <2 mm
c. <4 mm
d. <8 mm

Obstetrics / Assessment of Gestational Age

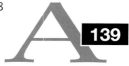

A. <6 mm.

The nuchal fold measurement is obtained between 15 and 20 weeks, and the nuchal fold should be less than 6 mm in thickness. A thickened (≥6 mm) nuchal fold can be an indicator of chromosomal abnormalities such as Down syndrome.

▶ Baun J: *Ob/Gyn Sonography: An Illustrated Review*. Pasadena, CA, Davies Publishing, 2016, p 278.

Which of the following best describes a normal value for nuchal translucency?

a. <2.5 mm
b. <3.5 mm
c. <4.5 mm
d. <5.5 mm

Obstetrics / Assessment of Gestational Age

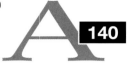 140

A. <2.5 mm.

Nuchal translucency (NT) is measured between 11 and 14 weeks, with a crown-rump length (CRL) no greater than 84 mm. Although the NT is dependent on gestational age, the maximal normal thickness is about 2.5 mm.

▶ Baun J: *Ob/Gyn Sonography: An Illustrated Review*. Pasadena, CA, Davies Publishing, 2016, pp 276–277.

281

Which of the following statements is the best definition of asymmetric intrauterine growth restriction (IUGR)?

a. All biometric parameters are proportionally small.
b. Some but not all fetal biometric measurements are reduced.
c. The fetus measures large for dates.
d. Asymmetric IUGR is the reduction of fetal body size.

Obstetrics / Complications

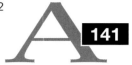

B. Some but not all fetal biometric measurements are reduced.

Asymmetric IUGR is characterized by the disproportionate reduction in some biometric growth parameters while others remain normal for gestational age. Typically, the abdominal circumference measures below the 10th percentile while the biparietal diameter (BPD), head circumference (HC), and femur length (FL) remain appropriate for dates. Asymmetric IUGR accounts for approximately 75% of IUGR cases.

▶ Baun J: *Ob/Gyn Sonography: An Illustrated Review*. Pasadena, CA, Davies Publishing, 2016, pp 305–306.

The fetal condition characterized by all biometric parameters measuring less than expected for a given gestational age is:

a. asymmetric intrauterine growth restriction
b. Beckwith-Wiedemann syndrome
c. symmetric intrauterine growth restriction
d. trisomy 21

Obstetrics / Complications

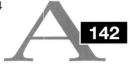

C. Symmetric intrauterine growth restriction.

Symmetric intrauterine growth restriction (IUGR) is present when all of the biometric parameters—biparietal diameter (BPD), head circumference (HC), abdominal circumference (AC), and femur length (FL)—are proportionally small for dates. Symmetric IUGR is more likely to be associated with congenital anomalies and genetic abnormalities than is asymmetric IUGR.

▶ Baun J: *Ob/Gyn Sonography: An Illustrated Review*. Pasadena, CA, Davies Publishing, 2016, p 305.

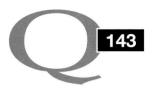

Symmetric intrauterine growth restriction (IUGR) may be associated with which of the following Doppler findings?

a. low-resistance middle cerebral artery
b. low-resistance umbilical artery
c. low-resistance ductus venosus
d. low-resistance renal artery

Obstetrics / Complications

A 143

A. Low-resistance middle cerebral artery.

With symmetric IUGR, there is usually increased resistance in the umbilical artery and decreased resistance in the middle cerebral artery. Although abnormal MCA Doppler would not be the sole indicator in identifying symmetric IUGR, it can assist in clinical decision making.

▶ Baun J: *Ob/Gyn Sonography: An Illustrated Review*. Pasadena, CA, Davies Publishing, 2016, p 304.

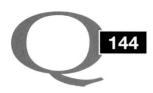

Q 144

A diamniotic/monochorionic pregnancy is suggested by a separating membrane that measures:

a. >2 mm
b. <2 mm
c. <4 mm
d. >4 mm

Obstetrics / Complications

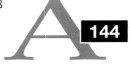

B. <2 mm.

A diamniotic/monochorionic gestation is one chorion (outer sac) with two amnions (inner sacs). The separating membrane is thin—only two layers thick (<2 mm). A separating membrane that measures more than 2 mm would indicate a dichorionic gestation.

- Baun J: *Ob/Gyn Sonography: An Illustrated Review*. Pasadena, CA, Davies Publishing, 2016, p 315.
- Gill KA: Multiple gestations and their complications. In Gill KA: *Ultrasound in Obstetrics and Gynecology: A Practitioner's Guide*. Pasadena, CA, Davies Publishing, 2014, p 295.

Which statement most accurately describes this image of a twin gestation?

a. The twins are diamniotic/monochorionic.
b. The twins are conjoined.
c. The twins are diamniotic/dichorionic.
d. The twins are growth discordant.

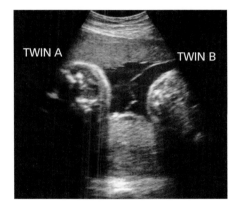

Obstetrics / Complications

A 145

C. The twins are diamniotic/dichorionic.

The correct answer is diamniotic/dichorionic because there are two placentas with a thick membrane. This twin gestation cannot be diamniotic/monochorionic because there is clearly one placenta anterior and one posterior. The twins cannot be conjoined because we see a separating membrane, and discordant growth is determined by fetal measurements.

▶ Baun J: *Ob/Gyn Sonography: An Illustrated Review*. Pasadena, CA, Davies Publishing, 2016, p 313.
▶ Gill KA: Multiple gestations and their complications. In Gill KA: *Ultrasound in Obstetrics and Gynecology: A Practitioner's Guide*. Pasadena, CA, Davies Publishing, 2014, pp 293–296.

The membrane separating these twins indicates what about this pregnancy?

a. It is diamniotic/monochorionic.
b. It is monoamniotic/dichorionic.
c. It is monoamniotic/monochorionic.
d. It is diamniotic/dichorionic.

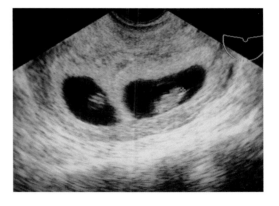

Obstetrics / Complications

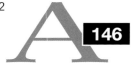

D. It is diamniotic/dichorionic.

This image is diagnostic of a diamniotic/dichorionic pregnancy as there are two clearly separate sacs separated by a thick membrane. With a diamniotic/monochorionic pregnancy, there would be one sac with a thin, almost invisible membrane separating the two fetuses. The first trimester is the best time to determine the type of multiple gestation present.

▶ Baun J: *Ob/Gyn Sonography: An Illustrated Review*. Pasadena, CA, Davies Publishing, 2016, p 313.
▶ Gill KA: Multiple gestations and their complications. In Gill KA: *Ultrasound in Obstetrics and Gynecology: A Practitioner's Guide*. Pasadena, CA, Davies Publishing, 2014, pp 293–296.

"Stuck twin" syndrome is associated with:

a. conjoined twins
b. twin-to-twin transfusion syndrome (TTTS)
c. twin reversed arterial perfusion (TRAP)
d. vanishing twin

Obstetrics / Complications

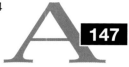

B. Twin-to-twin transfusion syndrome (TTTS).

Twin-to-twin transfusion syndrome is also called "poly-oligo" syndrome because while one twin is contained within a polyhydramniotic sac, the other is contained within an oligohydramniotic sac. *Stuck twin syndrome* is a severe form of this, in that the pump or donor twin's sac is so severely oligohydramniotic that its occupant appears "stuck" to the uterine wall. By contrast, *conjoined twins* share a single amniotic sac. *TRAP* refers to the acardiac twin malformation, and the *vanishing twin* condition occurs when one twin dies in the first trimester and is resorbed, resulting in delivery of a single fetus at term.

▶ Baun J: *Ob/Gyn Sonography: An Illustrated Review*. Pasadena, CA, Davies Publishing, 2016, pp 316–317.
▶ Gill KA: Multiple gestations and their complications. In Gill KA: *Ultrasound in Obstetrics and Gynecology: A Practitioner's Guide*. Pasadena, CA, Davies Publishing, 2014, p 300.

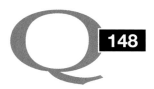

295

This image suggests a multiple gestation that is probably:

a. dizygotic
b. dichorionic
c. diamniotic
d. monoamniotic

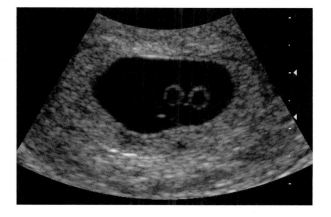

Obstetrics / Complications

A 148

C. Diamniotic.

This pregnancy is definitely monochorionic and the presence of two yolk sacs suggests diamnionicity. Many texts state that the number of yolk sacs is equivalent to the number of amnions present. In the literature, however, are documented cases of a single yolk sac with a diamniotic pregnancy. Therefore it is critical that transvaginal ultrasound be used to follow the pregnancy until a membrane is either confirmed or ruled out.

▶ Baun J: *Ob/Gyn Sonography: An Illustrated Review*. Pasadena, CA, Davies Publishing, 2016, p 313.

▶ Gill KA: Multiple gestations and their complications. In Gill KA: *Ultrasound in Obstetrics and Gynecology: A Practitioner's Guide*. Pasadena, CA, Davies Publishing, 2014, pp 293–294.

Twins that are connected to each other at the pelvic region would be termed:

a. pygopagus
b. craniopagus
c. thoracopagus
d. omphalopagus

Obstetrics / Complications

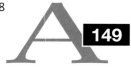

A. Pygopagus.

Pygopagus twins are conjoined twins that are connected at the pelvis. *Cranio* refers to the head, *thoraco* to the thorax, and *omphalo* to the abdomen.

- Baun J: *Ob/Gyn Sonography: An Illustrated Review*. Pasadena, CA, Davies Publishing, 2016, p 320.
- Gill KA: Multiple gestations and their complications. In Gill KA: *Ultrasound in Obstetrics and Gynecology: A Practitioner's Guide*. Pasadena, CA, Davies Publishing, 2014, pp 303, 305.

Twins' growth is considered discordant if:

a. their weights differ by more than 500 grams
b. their biparietal diameters differ by 2 mm
c. their abdominal circumferences differ by 5 mm
d. their cephalic indices are different

Obstetrics / Complications

A 150

A. Their weights differ by more than 500 grams.

Twins' growth is considered discordant when the sonographic estimates of their weights differ by more than 500 grams. A difference of a few millimeters between biometric measurements is not clinically significant. Twins' cephalic indices can vary for several reasons, and such variation is not necessarily an indicator of discordancy. Amniotic sacs can have different fluid levels for different reasons, which may not always indicate a growth discrepancy.

▶ Gill KA: Multiple gestations and their complications. In Gill KA: *Ultrasound in Obstetrics and Gynecology: A Practitioner's Guide*. Pasadena, CA, Davies Publishing, 2014, p 297.

151

A zygote that splits at 4–8 days at the inner-cell-mass stage results in which type of twinning?

a. monozygotic/monochorionic/diamniotic
b. dizygotic/dichorionic/diamniotic
c. monozygotic/dichorionic/diamniotic
d. monozygotic/monochorionic/monoamniotic

Obstetrics / Complications

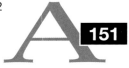

A. Monozygotic/monochorionic/diamniotic.

Monozygotic/monochorionic/diamniotic twin gestation is the most common type of monozygotic twinning. The inner cell mass divides at 4–8 days. Monozygotic twins that are dichorionic split before day 4. Monozygotic twins that are monoamniotic split between days 7 and 13. Dizygotic twins are the result of two separately fertilized ova and do not result from "splitting."

▶ Mehta TS: Multifetal pregnancy. In Rumack CM (ed): *Diagnostic Ultrasound*, 4th edition. St. Louis, Mosby, 2011, pp 1145–1165.

Q 152

A monochorionic/monoamniotic twin pregnancy will have:

a. two amnions and a single chorion
b. a single amnion and two chorions
c. two amnions and two chorions
d. a single amnion and a single chorion

Obstetrics / Complications

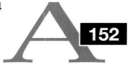

D. A single amnion and a single chorion.

Monochorionic means "having one chorion." *Monoamniotic* means "having one amnion." All monochorionic pregnancies result from a single fertilized ovum that splits, also known as *monozygotic twinning*. All monozygotic twins are identical.

▶ Baun J: *Ob/Gyn Sonography: An Illustrated Review*. Pasadena, CA, Davies Publishing, 2016, p 312.

Twin A appears in this image. Twin B, not imaged, appeared small and growth restricted. These findings are consistent with:

a. twin reversed arterial perfusion (TRAP) sequence

b. acardiac parabiotic twinning

c. twin-to-twin transfusion syndrome (TTTS)

d. twin embolization syndrome (TES)

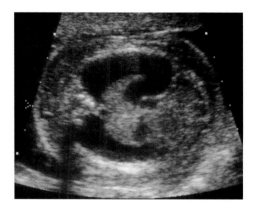

Obstetrics / Complications

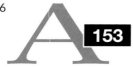

C. Twin-to-twin transfusion syndrome (TTTS).

This image of the fetal chest demonstrates signs of hydrops: pleural effusions and skin thickening. TTTS may occur in monochorionic twinning when one fetus is the "pump twin," sending blood to a plethoric recipient twin. The pump twin usually is found in an oligohydramniotic sac and is small, while the recipient is large, hydropic, and in a polyhydramniotic sac. By contrast, TES results from embolization of a deceased monochorionic twin to its co-twin. TRAP and acardiac parabiotic twinning occur when there is a pump twin that forms normally and a recipient twin with no heart or head.

- Baun J: *Ob/Gyn Sonography: An Illustrated Review*. Pasadena, CA, Davies Publishing, 2016, pp 316–317.
- Gill KA: Multiple gestations and their complications. In Gill KA: *Ultrasound in Obstetrics and Gynecology: A Practitioner's Guide*. Pasadena, CA, Davies Publishing, 2014, pp 299–300.

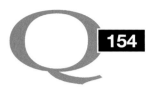

This transverse image demonstrates:

a. stuck twin
b. omphalocele
c. acardiacus
d. conjoined twins

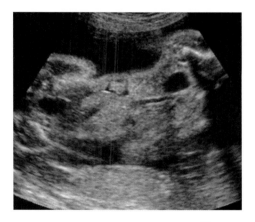

Obstetrics / Complications

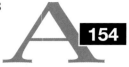

D. Conjoined twins.

This image demonstrates two fetal cross sections showing two urinary bladders with conjoined tissue in between. All conjoined twins are monozygotic and result from the zygote splitting after day 13.

▶ Baun J: *Ob/Gyn Sonography: An Illustrated Review*. Pasadena, CA, Davies Publishing, 2016, pp 320–321.

A twin gestation arising from two separately fertilized ova is called:

a. monoamniotic/dizygotic
b. diamniotic/monozygotic
c. dizygotic
d. monozygotic

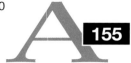

C. Dizygotic.

Dizygotic twins result from two separately fertilized ova, or zygotes. All dizygotic twins are fraternal, and all dizygotic twins are dichorionic/diamniotic. (By contrast, all monozygotic twins are identical.)

▶ Baun J: *Ob/Gyn Sonography: An Illustrated Review*. Pasadena, CA, Davies Publishing, 2016, p 313.

Which type of twinning does this image demonstrate?

a. monoamniotic/monochorionic
b. monoamniotic/dichorionic
c. diamniotic/monochorionic
d. diamniotic/dichorionic

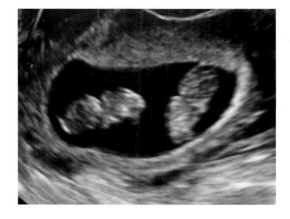

Obstetrics / Complications

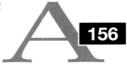

A. Monoamniotic/monochorionic.

This image is strongly suggestive of monoamniotic twins, since no membrane is visualized. However, the membrane in monochorionic/diamniotic twinning can be very thin and therefore very difficult to visualize, even with transvaginal ultrasound. As the management of monoamniotic and diamniotic pregnancies differs, a follow-up ultrasound should be performed to confirm absence of a membrane when monoamnionicity is suspected.

▶ Baun J: *Ob/Gyn Sonography: An Illustrated Review*. Pasadena, CA, Davies Publishing, 2016, pp 312–314.

157

Selective reduction of an embryo is also termed:

a. spontaneous abortion
b. incomplete abortion
c. inevitable abortion
d. therapeutic abortion

Obstetrics / Complications

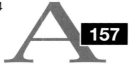

D. Therapeutic abortion.

A therapeutic abortion (TAB) is the same as an elective abortion or selective reduction. The term *selective reduction* is commonly used with higher-order multiple pregnancies in which one or more embryos are terminated in order to increase the chance of a successful pregnancy for the surviving fetuses.

▶ Baun J: *Ob/Gyn Sonography: An Illustrated Review*. Pasadena, CA, Davies Publishing, 2016, pp 320–321.
▶ Sliman MH, Gill KA: The first trimester. In Gill KA: *Ultrasound in Obstetrics and Gynecology: A Practitioner's Guide*. Pasadena, CA, Davies Publishing, 2014, p 105.

 **158**

The fetal anomaly most specifically associated with diabetes mellitus is:

a. prune belly syndrome
b. amniotic band sequence
c. clinodactyly
d. caudal regression syndrome

Obstetrics / Complications

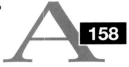

D. Caudal regression syndrome.

Although other congenital anomalies are also prevalent in patients with diabetes mellitus, caudal regression syndrome is 200–600 times more common in pregnancies of diabetic mothers. Caudal regression syndrome involves absence of the lower fetal spine and is associated with genitourinary anomalies, clubfeet, and other fetal abnormalities.

- Baun J: *Ob/Gyn Sonography: An Illustrated Review*. Pasadena, CA, Davies Publishing, 2016, p 158.
- Gill KA: Maternal disorders and pregnancy. In Gill KA: *Ultrasound in Obstetrics and Gynecology: A Practitioner's Guide*. Pasadena, CA, Davies Publishing, 2014, p 323.

Maternal blood pressure is considered elevated if it is:

a. >120/80 mmHg
b. >140/90 mmHg
c. >130/85 mmHg
d. >150/100 mmHg

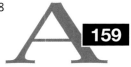

B. >140/90 mmHg.

Patients may have chronic hypertension, which is acquired prior to pregnancy, or have pregnancy-induced hypertension (PIH), acquired during the pregnancy. Blood pressure is elevated if it is above 140/90 mmHg.

- Baun J: *Ob/Gyn Sonography: An Illustrated Review*. Pasadena, CA, Davies Publishing, 2016, p 324.
- Gill KA: Maternal disorders and pregnancy. In Gill KA: *Ultrasound in Obstetrics and Gynecology: A Practitioner's Guide*. Pasadena, CA, Davies Publishing, 2014, p 314.

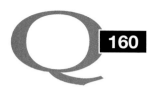

160

Which of these diabetic patients is most likely to have a fetus with severe anomalies?

a. gestational diabetic
b. type 2 diabetic
c. type 1 diabetic
d. class A diabetic

Obstetrics / Complications

C. Type 1 diabetic.

Although the fetuses of all diabetic mothers are at risk for anomalies, the offspring of pregestational diabetics are at significant risk because this type develops earlier in life and carries more significant complications, including circulatory complications, that affect fetal growth.

▶ Baun J: *Ob/Gyn Sonography: An Illustrated Review*. Pasadena, CA, Davies Publishing, 2016, pp 322–324.

▶ Gill KA: Maternal disorders and pregnancy. In Gill KA: *Ultrasound in Obstetrics and Gynecology: A Practitioner's Guide*. Pasadena, CA, Davies Publishing, 2014, p 319.

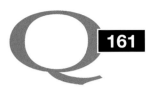

HELLP syndrome is a severe complication associated with:

a. pregnancy-induced hypertension
b. Rh isoimmunization
c. maternal gallbladder disease
d. fetal anemia

Obstetrics / Complications

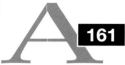

A. Pregnancy-induced hypertension.

HELLP, which stands for the symptoms that comprise this syndrome—hemolysis, elevated liver enzymes, and low platelets—is a potentially life-threatening complication of pregnancy-induced hypertension (PIH) and eclampsia.

▶ Gill KA: Maternal disorders and pregnancy. In Gill KA: *Ultrasound in Obstetrics and Gynecology: A Practitioner's Guide*. Pasadena, CA, Davies Publishing, 2014, pp 314–315.

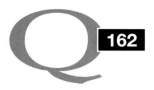

This image of a fetal pelvis depicts two anechoic structures, one of which is the fetal bladder. Findings from amniocentesis on this diabetic mother were normal. The diagnostic possibilities include which one of the following?

a. posterior urethral valves
b. anal atresia
c. cystic fibrosis
d. meconium ileus

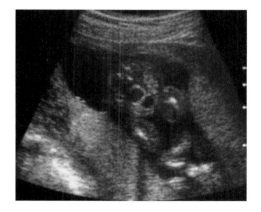

Obstetrics / Complications / AIT—PACSim

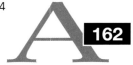

B. Anal atresia.

Anal atresia (a form of imperforate anus) is the result of arrested division of the cloaca in the urogenital sinus and rectum. It occurs in the 9th week of embryogenesis and there is a higher incidence among diabetics. Teratogens associated with this condition include alcohol and thalidomide. The prognosis is dependent on the associated anomalies, if any, and more than 95% of affected infants have successful function after postnatal surgical intervention.

▶ Baun J: *Ob/Gyn Sonography: An Illustrated Review*. Pasadena, CA, Davies Publishing, 2016, p 233.
▶ Gill KA: Anomalies associated with polyhydramnios. In Gill KA: *Ultrasound in Obstetrics and Gynecology: A Practitioner's Guide*. Pasadena, CA, Davies Publishing, 2014, p 325.

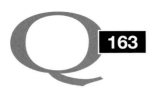

Of the following, which laboratory test will determine maternal glycemic control?

a. beta-hCG
b. CEA
c. MSAFP
d. Hgb A1C

Obstetrics / Complications

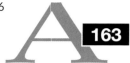

D. Hgb A1C.

Hemoglobin A1C (Hgb A1C) is a blood test that provides information on glucose control in diabetics. Human chorionic gonadotropin, beta subgroup (beta-hCG) and maternal serum alpha-fetoprotein (MSAFP) determine whether a pregnancy is present. Carcinoembryonic antigen (CEA) is a cancer-screening test.

▶ Gill KA: Maternal disorders and pregnancy. In Gill KA: *Ultrasound in Obstetrics and Gynecology: A Practitioner's Guide*. Pasadena, CA, Davies Publishing, 2014, p 326.

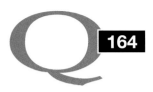

164

The placenta of a gestational diabetic is often edematous. The placental thickness at term should not exceed:

a. 4–5 cm
b. 2–3 cm
c. 3–4 cm
d. 5–6 cm

Obstetrics / Complications

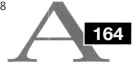

A. 4–5 cm.

The placenta is usually less than 4–5 cm in thickness during pregnancy. The maximum normal thickness at 20 weeks is 2–3 cm.

- Baun J: *Ob/Gyn Sonography: An Illustrated Review*. Pasadena, CA, Davies Publishing, 2016, p 36.
- Gill KA: Maternal disorders and pregnancy. In Gill KA: *Ultrasound in Obstetrics and Gynecology: A Practitioner's Guide*. Pasadena, CA, Davies Publishing, 2014, p 321.

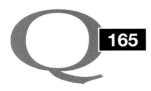

165

What is the term for excessive accumulation of fluid in at least two anatomic locations in the fetus?

a. anasarca
b. hydrops fetalis
c. ascites
d. hydrocephalus

Obstetrics / Complications

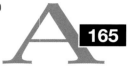

B. Hydrops fetalis.

Hydrops fetalis (fetal hydrops) is defined as two or more abnormal serous fluid collections in the fetus, which may include pleural effusions, abdominal ascites, and/or anasarca. Hydrops can lead to a cascade of fetal symptoms resulting from immune and nonimmune maternal issues. *Anasarca*—generalized edema of the skin—is simply one of them; *ascites*, fluid in the abdomen, is another symptom. *Hydrocephalus* is fluid within the ventricles of the brain and is not directly related to hydrops.

▶ Baun J: *Ob/Gyn Sonography: An Illustrated Review*. Pasadena, CA, Davies Publishing, 2016, p 302.

Of the following, which is a cause of immune hydrops?

a. diabetes
b. pregnancy-induced hypertension
c. TORCH infections
d. Rhesus (Rh) incompatibility

Obstetrics / Complications

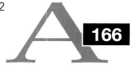

D. Rhesus (Rh) incompatibility.

Rh incompatibility is one cause of *immune* hydrops. Immune hydrops is fetal hydrops caused by antibodies the mother has developed that result in fetal anemia; most cases are caused by blood group incompatibilities. All other choices are causes of *nonimmune* hydrops.

▶ Baun J: *Ob/Gyn Sonography: An Illustrated Review*. Pasadena, CA, Davies Publishing, 2016, p 302.
▶ Gill KA: Maternal disorders and pregnancy. In Gill KA: *Ultrasound in Obstetrics and Gynecology: A Practitioner's Guide*. Pasadena, CA, Davies Publishing, 2014, p 318.

Q 167

Erythroblastosis fetalis is caused by:

a. Rh-negative father, Rh-negative mother, Rh-negative fetus
b. Rh-positive father, Rh-positive mother, Rh-negative fetus
c. Rh-positive father, Rh-negative mother, Rh-positive fetus
d. Rh-negative father, Rh-positive mother, Rh-positive fetus

Obstetrics / Complications

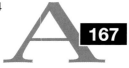

C. Rh-positive father, Rh-negative mother, Rh-positive fetus.

An Rh-positive father with an Rh-negative mother and an Rh-positive fetus leads to maternal isoimmunization from the Rh-positive fetal blood. The maternal antibodies can then cross the placental barrier and cause hemolytic disease in the fetus, leading to fetal hydrops. The maternal antibodies are sensitized during the first pregnancy, but it is not until the second pregnancy that fetal problems related to Rh isoimmunization will occur.

▶ Baun J: *Ob/Gyn Sonography: An Illustrated Review*. Pasadena, CA, Davies Publishing, 2016, p 302.
▶ Gill KA: Maternal disorders and pregnancy. In Gill KA: *Ultrasound in Obstetrics and Gynecology: A Practitioner's Guide*. Pasadena, CA, Davies Publishing, 2014, p 318.

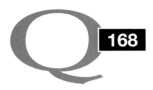 **168**

What is the term for the sonographic demonstration of intact fetal membranes protruding into the endocervical canal?

a. engorgement
b. premature rupture of membranes (PROM)
c. funneling
d. preterm labor

Obstetrics / Complications

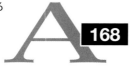

C. Funneling.

Funneling implies protrusion of the membranes into a dilated endocervical canal; it can be a false-positive finding with both transabdominal and transvaginal sonography due to, respectively, bladder distention and lower-uterine-segment contractions. *PROM* and *preterm labor* may occur with or without cervical dilatation.

▶ Foy PM: Ultrasound of the cervix during pregnancy. In Gill KA: *Ultrasound in Obstetrics and Gynecology: A Practitioner's Guide*. Pasadena, CA, Davies Publishing, 2014, p 217.

The primary sonographic sign observed in premature rupture of membranes (PROM) is:

a. oligohydramnios
b. polyhydramnios
c. cord prolapse
d. respiratory distress syndrome

Obstetrics / Complications

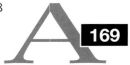

A. Oligohydramnios.

PROM is a common cause of oligohydramnios. Leakage of fluid through the vagina will cause continued oligohydramnios if the membranes do not reseal.

- Baun J: *Ob/Gyn Sonography: An Illustrated Review*. Pasadena, CA, Davies Publishing, 2016, p 331.
- Drose JA: Multiple gestations. In Raatz Stephenson S (ed): *Diagnostic Medical Sonography: Obstetrics and Gynecology*, 3rd edition. Philadelphia, Lippincott Williams & Wilkins, 2012, ch 26.
- Rodriguez J, Gill KA: Anomalies associated with oligohydramnios. In Gill KA: *Ultrasound in Obstetrics and Gynecology: A Practitioner's Guide*. Pasadena, CA, Davies Publishing, 2014, pp 269, 283, 284.

339

Preterm labor may be caused by:

a. placenta previa
b. subserosal fibroid
c. polyhydramnios
d. hypothyroidism

Obstetrics / Complications

A 170

C. Polyhydramnios.

Overdistention of the uterus leads to contractions, causing preterm labor.

▶ Baun J: *Ob/Gyn Sonography: An Illustrated Review*. Pasadena, CA, Davies Publishing, 2016, p 331.
▶ Drose JA: Multiple gestations. In Raatz Stephenson S (ed): *Diagnostic Medical Sonography: Obstetrics and Gynecology*, 3rd edition. Philadelphia, Lippincott Williams & Wilkins, 2012, ch 26.

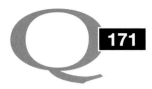

341

This patient is at high risk for:

a. bleeding
b. amniotic fluid embolus
c. ectopic pregnancy
d. preterm birth

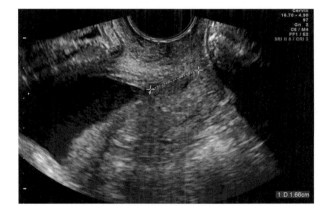

Obstetrics / Complications

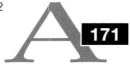

D. Preterm birth.

The length of the cervix should measure 25 mm or greater. This cervix measures 16.6 mm, which is considered shortened. This patient is at high risk for preterm labor.

- Baun J: *Ob/Gyn Sonography: An Illustrated Review*. Pasadena, CA, Davies Publishing, 2016, p 331.
- Foy PM: Ultrasound of the cervix during pregnancy. In Gill KA: *Ultrasound in Obstetrics and Gynecology: A Practitioner's Guide*. Pasadena, CA, Davies Publishing, 2014, pp 216–217.

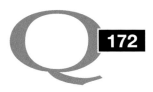

343

The sonographic findings demonstrated in this image of the fetal chest are consistent with a fetus affected by:

a. intrauterine growth restriction (IUGR)
b. maternal hypertension
c. stuck twin syndrome
d. Rh isoimmunization

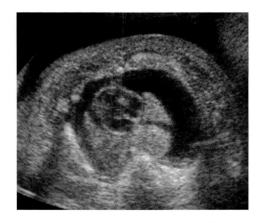

Obstetrics / Complications

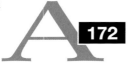

D. Rh isoimmunization.

This image of the fetal chest is consistent with fetal hydrops. Note the marked skin thickening and pleural effusions. In this image the heart is of normal size, although with Rh isoimmunization heart failure with cardiomegaly may occur, along with other abnormalities.

▶ Baun J: *Ob/Gyn Sonography: An Illustrated Review*. Pasadena, CA, Davies Publishing, 2016, p 302.

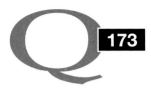

345

In which situation would a fetal shunt procedure be indicated?

a. hydranencephaly
b. pleural effusion
c. polycystic kidneys
d. duodenal atresia

Obstetrics / Complications

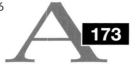

B. Pleural effusion.

Severe pleural effusions cause compression of the lung tissue. A shunt can be placed into the fetal chest under ultrasound guidance, allowing the pleural effusion to drain into the amniotic fluid. Intrauterine shunt placement is not currently used for hydranencephaly, polycystic kidneys, or duodenal atresia.

- Baun J: *Ob/Gyn Sonography: An Illustrated Review*. Pasadena, CA, Davies Publishing, 2016, p 472.
- Oshiro BT, Gill KA: Invasive procedures. In Gill KA: *Ultrasound in Obstetrics and Gynecology: A Practitioner's Guide*. Pasadena, CA, Davies Publishing, 2014, p 451.

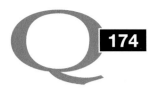 **174**

Which procedure is used to treat massive polyhydramnios?

a. therapeutic amnioreduction
b. percutaneous umbilical blood sampling
c. pleuroamniotic shunting
d. intrapartum amniotransfusion

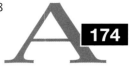

A. Therapeutic amnioreduction.

Severe polyhydramnios increases the risk of preterm labor due to uterine distention and induces maternal breathing problems. When severe polyhydramnios is present, a therapeutic amnioreduction can be performed whereby some of the amniotic fluid is withdrawn and discarded. There is a risk of premature rupture of membranes or preterm labor, as there is with any invasive procedure.

- Baun J: *Ob/Gyn Sonography: An Illustrated Review*. Pasadena, CA, Davies Publishing, 2016, p 472.
- Oshiro BT, Gill KA: Invasive procedures. In Gill KA: *Ultrasound in Obstetrics and Gynecology: A Practitioner's Guide*. Pasadena, CA, Davies Publishing, 2014, pp 446–447.

175

A postpartum complication that may follow cesarean section is:

a. pregnancy-induced hypertensive disorder
b. bladder flap hematoma
c. hyperemesis gravidarum
d. supine hypotensive syndrome

Obstetrics / Complications / AIT—PACSim

A **175**

B. Bladder flap hematoma.

Bladder flap hematoma is a sonographically complex mass located between the uterus and the bladder. It may be seen after c-section delivery.

▶ Baun J: *Ob/Gyn Sonography: An Illustrated Review*. Pasadena, CA, Davies Publishing, 2016, pp 334–335.

▶ Shatterly D: The postpartum uterus. In Raatz Stephenson S (ed): *Diagnostic Medical Sonography: Obstetrics and Gynecology*, 3rd edition. Philadelphia, Lippincott Williams & Wilkins, 2012, ch 30.

A febrile patient presents for a pelvic sonogram three days after undergoing cesarean section. Sonography reveals echogenic and anechoic areas within the endometrial cavity. These findings are most consistent with:

a. adenomyosis
b. retained products of conception
c. bladder flap hematoma
d. retained intrauterine contraceptive device

Obstetrics / Complications

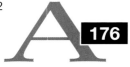

B. Retained products of conception.

A patient with bleeding, pain, and/or fever after delivery should be evaluated sonographically for retained placenta. Adenomyosis is not likely to be visualized immediately postpartum. Bladder flap hematoma is a possibility after c-section but does not present as abnormalities within the endometrial canal.

- Baun J: *Ob/Gyn Sonography: An Illustrated Review*. Pasadena, CA, Davies Publishing, 2016, pp 332–333, 453.
- Shatterly D: The postpartum uterus. In Raatz Stephenson S (ed): *Diagnostic Medical Sonography: Obstetrics and Gynecology*, 3rd edition. Philadelphia, Lippincott Williams & Wilkins, 2012, ch 30.

A common cause of acute primary postpartum hemorrhage is:

a. uterine atony
b. retained products of conception
c. endometriosis
d. retained umbilical cord

Obstetrics / Complications

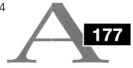

A. Uterine atony.

Uterine atony results from weakened uterine muscles from multiple gestation, polyhydramnios, and/or a large fetus. Delayed hemorrhage is more likely the result of retention of products of conception.

▶ Baun J: *Ob/Gyn Sonography: An Illustrated Review*. Pasadena, CA, Davies Publishing, 2016, p 332.
▶ Shatterly D: The postpartum uterus. In Raatz Stephenson S (ed): *Diagnostic Medical Sonography: Obstetrics and Gynecology*, 3rd edition. Philadelphia, Lippincott Williams & Wilkins, 2012, ch 30.

178

Which statement best characterizes the amniotic fluid index (AFI)?

a. It is a qualitative means of calculating amniotic fluid.
b. It is a quantitative means of calculating amniotic fluid.
c. It is a method for performing an amniocentesis.
d. It is not a reliable method for evaluating amniotic fluid levels.

Obstetrics / Amniotic Fluid

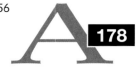

B. It is a quantitative means of calculating amniotic fluid.

"Eyeballing" fluid levels is a qualitative means of evaluating amniotic fluid used by experienced practitioners. The AFI is an accepted practice and is considered reliable. Although an adequate fluid pocket is necessary for amniocentesis, the AFI is not a method for performing the procedure.

- Baun J: *Ob/Gyn Sonography: An Illustrated Review*. Pasadena, CA, Davies Publishing, 2016, pp 153–154.
- Rodriguez J, Gill KA: Anomalies associated with oligohydramnios. In Gill KA: *Ultrasound in Obstetrics and Gynecology: A Practitioner's Guide*. Pasadena, CA, Davies Publishing, 2014, p 286.

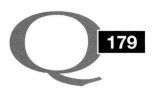

357

How is the amniotic fluid index (AFI) acquired?

a. subjective analysis
b. summation of the measurement of two horizontal pockets
c. summation of measurements of the single deepest pocket in each uterine quadrant free of fetal parts
d. measurement of the single deepest pocket

Obstetrics / Amniotic Fluid

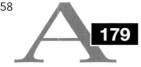

C. Summation of measurements of the single deepest pocket in each uterine quadrant free of fetal parts.

In a singleton pregnancy, the standard AFI is performed by measuring the deepest pocket of fluid (void of fetal parts) in each of four quadrants perpendicular to the uterus; these measurements are then added. In a multiple pregnancy, the deepest vertical pocket (also called the *maximum vertical pocket* or *single deepest pocket*) of fluid for each fetus is used.

▶ Baun J: *Ob/Gyn Sonography: An Illustrated Review*. Pasadena, CA, Davies Publishing, 2016, pp 153–154.
▶ Rodriguez J, Gill KA: The second and third trimesters: basic and targeted scans. In Gill KA: *Ultrasound in Obstetrics and Gynecology: A Practitioner's Guide*. Pasadena, CA, Davies Publishing, 2014, pp 138–139.

This sonogram in a trisomy 18 male fetus with abnormal flexion of the arms demonstrates:

a. polyhydramnios
b. normal amniotic fluid volume
c. anhydramnios
d. oligohydramnios

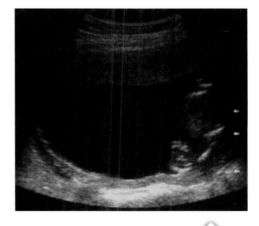

Obstetrics / Amniotic Fluid

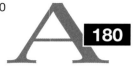

A. Polyhydramnios.

Polyhydramnios is seen in association with many fetal anomalies, especially those in which fetal swallowing is impaired.

- Baun J: *Ob/Gyn Sonography: An Illustrated Review*. Pasadena, CA, Davies Publishing, 2016, p 154.
- Gill KA: Anomalies associated with polyhydramnios. In Gill KA: *Ultrasound in Obstetrics and Gynecology: A Practitioner's Guide*. Pasadena, CA, Davies Publishing, 2014, p 230.

361

What is the single-deepest-pocket measurement of amniotic fluid that indicates polyhydramnios?

a. >12 cm
b. >8 cm
c. >14 cm
d. >16 cm

Obstetrics / Amniotic Fluid

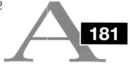

B. >8 cm.

If the single deepest pocket is greater than 80 mm (8 cm), polyhydramnios is present.

- Baun J: *Ob/Gyn Sonography: An Illustrated Review*. Pasadena, CA, Davies Publishing, 2016, pp 230, 249–251.
- Gill KA: *Ultrasound in Obstetrics and Gynecology: A Practitioner's Guide*. Pasadena, CA, Davies Publishing, 2014, p 154.

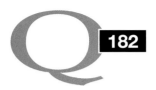

This transverse image of a fetal head in a patient with oligohydramnios demonstrates:

a. increased nuchal fold thickness
b. abnormal cerebellum
c. Spalding's sign
d. choroid plexus cysts

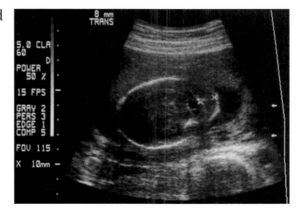

Obstetrics / Amniotic Fluid

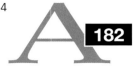

A. Increased nuchal fold thickness.

This image demonstrates a thickened nuchal fold. In this image the nuchal fold measures 10 mm, which exceeds the normal size of 6 mm or less. Oligohydramnios may be associated with chromosomal anomalies, so this pregnancy raises a concern for trisomy 21 (Down syndrome). Spalding's sign is the appearance of collapsed fetal cranial bones associated with fetal demise.

- Baun J: *Ob/Gyn Sonography: An Illustrated Review*. Pasadena, CA, Davies Publishing, 2016, p 278.
- Rodriguez J, Gill KA: Anomalies associated with oligohydramnios. In Gill KA: *Ultrasound in Obstetrics and Gynecology: A Practitioner's Guide*. Pasadena, CA, Davies Publishing, 2014, p 354.

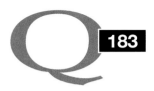

This image displays a major complication associated with renal agenesis that leads to fatal pulmonary hypoplasia in the fetus at birth. What finding is present in this image?

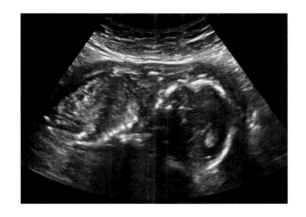

a. polyhydramnios
b. anhydramnios
c. oligohydramnios
d. amniotic fluid embolus

Obstetrics / Amniotic Fluid

A **183**

B. Anhydramnios.

This image presents a fetus with bilateral renal agenesis and anhydramnios. These conditions are unfortunately 100% fatal to the fetus because of the severe pulmonary hypoplasia that results. Fluid infusion can be performed to aid in the diagnosis of renal agenesis because the exam is more difficult without amniotic fluid, but the condition is still lethal.

▶ Baun J: *Ob/Gyn Sonography: An Illustrated Review*. Pasadena, CA, Davies Publishing, 2016, pp 155, 252–253.

367

Fetal lung maturity is most commonly and most accurately assessed by:

a. placental grading
b. comparing fetal lung to liver echogenicity
c. amniocentesis
d. observing fetal breathing movements

Obstetrics / Amniotic Fluid

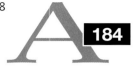

C. Amniocentesis.

Amniocentesis used to determine lung maturity measures the ratio of lecithin to sphingomyelin in amniotic fluid. An L/S ratio greater than 2.0 correlates with fetal lung maturity. Placental grading, fetal breathing, and fetal lung echogenicity have no bearing on lung maturity.

▶ Baun J: *Ob/Gyn Sonography: An Illustrated Review*. Pasadena, CA, Davies Publishing, 2016, pp 153, 155, 275–276.
▶ Magner RG Jr, Vance CA: Ultrasound of the normal fetal chest. abdomen, and pelvis. In Raatz Stephenson S (ed): *Diagnostic Medical Sonography: Obstetrics and Gynecology*, 3rd edition. Philadelphia, Lippincott Williams & Wilkins, 2012, ch 20.

Q 185

What is the most serious risk to the fetus with anhydramnios for an extended period of time?

a. pulmonary hypoplasia
b. cardiac failure
c. limb abnormalities
d. cleft lip

Obstetrics / Amniotic Fluid

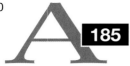

A. Pulmonary hypoplasia.

Amniotic fluid is essential to allow fetal lungs to mature. Without the fetus "breathing in" amniotic fluid throughout the pregnancy, there will be pulmonary hypoplasia at birth, which can be fatal.

- Baun J: *Ob/Gyn Sonography: An Illustrated Review*. Pasadena, CA, Davies Publishing, 2016, pp 166–167.
- Oshiro BT, Gill KA: Invasive procedures. In Gill KA: *Ultrasound in Obstetrics and Gynecology: A Practitioner's Guide*. Pasadena, CA, Davies Publishing, 2014, p 451.

An abnormal decrease in maternal serum alpha-fetoprotein (MSAFP) may be found in cases of:

a. spina bifida
b. omphalocele
c. trisomy 21
d. multiple gestations

Obstetrics / Genetic Studies

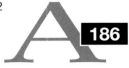

C. Trisomy 21.

Low MSAFP may be seen in the presence of trisomy 21. Elevated MSAFP, by comparison, is seen with open neural tube defects and open ventral wall defects.

▶ Baun J: *Ob/Gyn Sonography: An Illustrated Review*. Pasadena, CA, Davies Publishing, 2016, pp 273–274.

187

Which of the following maternal serum markers is typically measured to screen for fetal anomalies?

a. serum bilirubin
b. acetylcholinesterase
c. progesterone
d. alpha-fetoprotein

Obstetrics / Genetic Studies

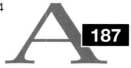

D. Alpha-fetoprotein.

Multiple marker screening (MMS)—which may include screening for maternal alpha-fetoprotein (MSAFP), estriol, and human chorionic gonadotropin (hCG)—is done between 15 and 22 weeks' gestation. Based on the results of the MMS, the risk for aneuploidy and certain fetal malformations is calculated utilizing the maternal age and menstrual age. Although MMS is quickly being replaced by first trimester cell-free DNA testing, MMS is still routinely performed to screen for aneuploidy.

▶ Baun J: *Ob/Gyn Sonography: An Illustrated Review*. Pasadena, CA, Davies Publishing, 2016, pp 272–273.
▶ Johnson JM: Overview of obstetric sonography. In Rumack CM (ed): *Diagnostic Ultrasound*, 4th edition. St. Louis, Mosby, 2011, pp 961–974.

188

What is the best definition of *tenting*?

a. proliferation of placental tissue between the amnions in a twin pregnancy
b. discoloration of amniotic fluid when blue dye is introduced
c. elevation of the amnion by a needle when the membranes have not fused
d. use of a stent with a triangular tip

Obstetrics / Genetic Studies

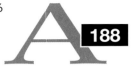

C. Elevation of the amnion by a needle when the membranes have not fused.

Sometimes the amniocentesis needle does not penetrate the amnion—the needle pushes the amnion but does not pierce it. This is called *tenting* and is more common when amniocentesis is conducted earlier rather than later in the period during which the procedure can be performed (15–20 weeks' gestation).

▶ Oshiro BT, Gill KA: Invasive procedures. In Gill KA: *Ultrasound in Obstetrics and Gynecology: A Practitioner's Guide*. Pasadena, CA, Davies Publishing, 2014, p 452.

Q 189

The key role of sonography in performing amniocentesis is to:

a. identify abnormal biochemical markers
b. detect chromosomal abnormalities
c. check for neural tube defects
d. localize placental and fetal position

Obstetrics / Genetic Studies

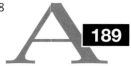

D. Localize placental and fetal position.

The other choices may be indications that amniocentesis should be performed, but the role of sonography in the actual performance of the procedure is to locate the fetus and placenta to aid in safe guidance of the needle. Ultrasound should be used to document fetal heart rate before and after the procedure.

▶ Baun J: *Ob/Gyn Sonography: An Illustrated Review*. Pasadena, CA, Davies Publishing, 2016, pp 275–276.
▶ Johnson JM: Ultrasound-guided invasive fetal procedures. In Rumack CM (ed): *Diagnostic Ultrasound*, 4th edition. St. Louis, Mosby, 2011, pp 1543–1557.

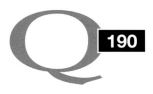

The most important advantage of chorionic villus sampling over amniocentesis is:

a. less risk of miscarriage than amniocentesis
b. earlier diagnosis of chromosomal abnormalities
c. less chance of bleeding following the procedure
d. less risk of placental separation

Obstetrics / Genetic Studies

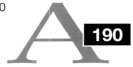

B. Earlier diagnosis of chromosomal abnormalities.

Because it can be performed in the first trimester—sooner than amniocentesis is performed—chorionic villus sampling (CVS) allows decisions to be made earlier regarding continuing the pregnancy in the event of chromosomal abnormality.

- Baun J: *Ob/Gyn Sonography: An Illustrated Review*. Pasadena, CA, Davies Publishing, 2016, pp 274–275.
- Johnson JM: Ultrasound-guided invasive fetal procedures. In Rumack CM (ed): *Diagnostic Ultrasound*, 4th edition. St. Louis, Mosby, 2011, pp 1543–1557.

191

Chorionic villus sampling (CVS) is best performed at:

a. 4–6 weeks
b. 14–16 weeks
c. 16–18 weeks
d. 10–13 weeks

Obstetrics / Genetic Studies

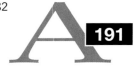

D. 10–13 weeks.

CVS is usually performed between 10 and 13 weeks—earlier than amniocentesis can be safely performed (15–20 weeks). CVS at 4–6 weeks is too early for cells to grow out of the specimen. After 14 weeks amniocentesis can be performed.

- Baun J: *Ob/Gyn Sonography: An Illustrated Review*. Pasadena, CA, Davies Publishing, 2016, pp 274–275.
- Callen PW: *Ultrasonography in Obstetrics and Gynecology*, 5th edition. Philadelphia, Elsevier, 2008, p 67.
- Gill KA: Fetal syndromes. In Gill KA: *Ultrasound in Obstetrics and Gynecology: A Practitioner's Guide*. Pasadena, CA, Davies Publishing, 2014, p 339.

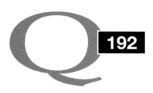

Which of the following chorionic villus sampling (CVS) methods is similar in technique to an amniocentesis?

a. transvaginal
b. transabdominal
c. intravenous
d. transvesical

Obstetrics / Genetic Studies

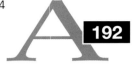

B. Transabdominal.

The transabdominal CVS method is similar in technique to amniocentesis, except that the needle is advanced only to the level of the placenta and not into the amniotic sac. With the transcervical approach a catheter is inserted into the cervix and suction is used to sample the chorionic villi.

- Baun J: *Ob/Gyn Sonography: An Illustrated Review*. Pasadena, CA, Davies Publishing, 2016, pp 274–276.
- Oshiro BT, Gill KA: Invasive procedures. In Gill KA: *Ultrasound in Obstetrics and Gynecology: A Practitioner's Guide*. Pasadena, CA, Davies Publishing, 2014, pp 445–446.

385

Which term denotes a congenital condition created when each parent contributes a defective copy of a gene?

a. autosomal recessive
b. aneuploidy
c. trisomy
d. autosomal dominant

Obstetrics / Genetic Studies

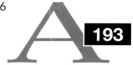

A. Autosomal recessive.

In *autosomal recessive diseases* each parent must pass on a defective copy of the gene or the fetus will be unaffected. In *autosomal dominant conditions* only one parent needs to contribute the gene for the fetus to have the condition. *Aneuploidy* is a generic term for an abnormal number of chromosomes, and *trisomy* denotes three copies of a chromosome.

▶ Baun J: *Ob/Gyn Sonography: An Illustrated Review*. Pasadena, CA, Davies Publishing, 2016, p 282.

What is the probability that disorders inherited in an autosomal recessive fashion will be passed on to offspring?

a. 50%

b. 75%

c. 100%

d. 25%

Obstetrics / Genetic Studies

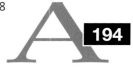

D. 25%.

In autosomal recessive disorders, in which both parents must pass on a defective copy of a gene, the fetus has a 25% chance of inheriting the disorder (i.e., since each parent has a 50% chance, the chance of both passing on the recessive gene is reduced to 25%). Autosomal dominant disorders carry a 50% chance of being passed on to offspring (since a dominant gene will express itself if it is inherited from only one parent).

- Baun J: *Ob/Gyn Sonography: An Illustrated Review*. Pasadena, CA, Davies Publishing, 2016, p 282.
- Gill KA: Fetal syndromes. In Gill KA: *Ultrasound in Obstetrics and Gynecology: A Practitioner's Guide*. Pasadena, CA, Davies Publishing, 2014, p 335.

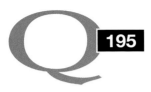

195

A congenital condition characterized by the presence of three chromosomes instead of the normal two is called:

a. disomy
b. monosomy
c. trisomy
d. tetrasomy

Obstetrics / Genetic Studies

A 195

C. Trisomy.

With the exception of the sex chromosomes, normal chromosomes are in duplicate. Trisomy occurs when a chromosome is in triplicate, meaning that there are three copies of one chromosome. Common trisomies are Down syndrome (trisomy 21) and Edwards syndrome (trisomy 18).

Baun J: *Ob/Gyn Sonography: An Illustrated Review*. Pasadena, CA, Davies Publishing, 2016, p 282.

How long after demise does general fetal maceration usually become sonographically apparent?

a. 24 hours
b. 10–14 days
c. 4 days
d. 1 month

Obstetrics / Fetal Demise

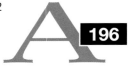

B. 10–14 days.

Although the process of maceration begins immediately, it does so in a sterile environment and usually does not become sonographically apparent for 10 to 14 days following fetal demise.

▶ Rodriguez J, Gill KA: Anomalies associated with oligohydramnios. In Gill KA: *Ultrasound in Obstetrics and Gynecology: A Practitioner's Guide*. Pasadena, CA, Davies Publishing, 2014, pp 270–271.

393

197

After fetal demise, gas can sometimes be seen in the fetal chest and/or abdomen due to breakdown of fetal tissues. This is called:

a. Robert's sign
b. Spalding's sign
c. Murphy's sign
d. Deuel's sign

Obstetrics / Fetal Demise

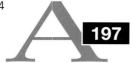

A. Robert's sign.

Robert's sign is the appearance of gas in the fetal chest and/or abdomen following fetal demise. *Spalding's sign* refers to collapse and overlapping of cranial bones, *Murphy's sign* refers to gallbladder pain when pressure is applied across the gallbladder region, and *Deuel's sign* (the halo sign) is a radiographic finding of fetal demise.

▶ Rodriguez J, Gill KA: Anomalies associated with oligohydramnios. In Gill KA: *Ultrasound in Obstetrics and Gynecology: A Practitioner's Guide*. Pasadena, CA, Davies Publishing, 2014, pp 270–271.

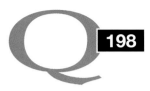

Overlapping of the fetal cranial bones that may accompany fetal demise is termed:

a. dolichocephaly
b. Spalding's sign
c. brachycephaly
d. anencephaly

Obstetrics / Fetal Demise

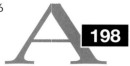

B. Spalding's sign.

Spalding's sign is the sonographic visualization of overlapping cranial bones secondary to fetal demise. In addition, the head usually appears flattened. *Anencephaly* is absence of the fetal head, although the fetus may be alive in utero, and both *dolichocephaly* and *brachycephaly* are head shapes not specifically associated with fetal death.

▶ Baun J: *Ob/Gyn Sonography: An Illustrated Review*. Pasadena, CA, Davies Publishing, 2016, p 311.

a. Dandy-Walker malformation
b. Arnold-Chiari II
c. alobar holoprosencephaly
d. ventriculomegaly

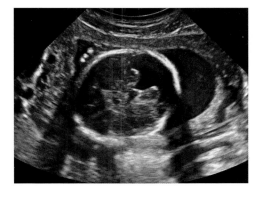

Obstetrics / Fetal Abnormalities

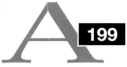

A. Dandy-Walker malformation.

This image demonstrates findings consistent with Dandy-Walker malformation, including a large cisterna magna cyst communicating with the fourth ventricle and absent cerebellar vermis. With Arnold-Chiari II the cisterna magna is obliterated. Alobar holoprosencephaly is ruled out because of the presence of a falx cerebri. Ventriculomegaly is not seen in this image.

- Baun J: *Ob/Gyn Sonography: An Illustrated Review*. Pasadena, CA, Davies Publishing, 2016, p 129.
- Gill KA: Anomalies associated with polyhydramnios. In Gill KA: *Ultrasound in Obstetrics and Gynecology: A Practitioner's Guide*. Pasadena, CA, Davies Publishing, 2014, pp 235–236.

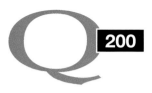

399

Alobar, semilobar, and lobar are three types of:

a. encephalocele
b. congenital pulmonary airway malformation (CPAM)
c. holoprosencephaly
d. congenital diaphragmatic hernia (CDH)

Obstetrics / Fetal Abnormalities

A 200

C. Holoprosencephaly.

Holoprosencephaly is a midline cranial defect that affects the brain and/or face and can be ranked, in order of most severe to least severe, as alobar, semilobar, or lobar. *Encephalocele* is protrusion of fetal meninges and/or brain from a cranial defect. *CPAM* is a mass in the fetal chest. *CDH* is protrusion of abdominal contents into the fetal thorax.

▶ Baun J: *Ob/Gyn Sonography: An Illustrated Review*. Pasadena, CA, Davies Publishing, 2016, pp 126–128.
▶ Gill KA: Anomalies associated with polyhydramnios. In Gill KA: *Ultrasound in Obstetrics and Gynecology: A Practitioner's Guide*. Pasadena, CA, Davies Publishing, 2014, pp 238–239.

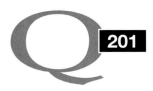

Holoprosencephaly is often associated with:

a. trisomy 18
b. trisomy 21
c. triploidy
d. trisomy 13

Obstetrics / Fetal Abnormalities

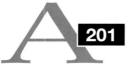

D. Trisomy 13.

Holoprosencephaly may be seen in euploid fetuses, especially in its least severe (lobar) form, but alobar holoprosencephaly is commonly associated with trisomy 13, a lethal syndrome. In addition to the monoventricle common with alobar holoprosencephaly, sonographically visible anomalies usually include severe midline facial clefts, a single orbit, and a supraorbital proboscis with a single nostril (*cebocephaly*).

▶ Baun J: *Ob/Gyn Sonography: An Illustrated Review*. Pasadena, CA, Davies Publishing, 2016, p 128.
▶ Gill KA: Fetal syndromes. In Gill KA: *Ultrasound in Obstetrics and Gynecology: A Practitioner's Guide*. Pasadena, CA, Davies Publishing, 2014, pp 348–349.

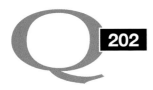

This image of the fetal head demonstrates:

a. small orbital diameters
b. choroid plexus cysts
c. bilateral hydrocephalus
d. normal ventricular atria

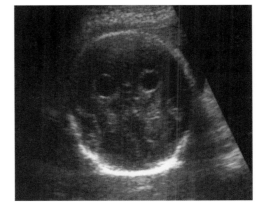

Obstetrics / Fetal Abnormalities

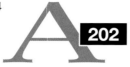

B. Choroid plexus cysts.

Choroid plexus cysts are a common finding and, when isolated, are of no clinical significance. If choroid plexus cysts are found with other signs of aneuploidy, though, further investigation is warranted. Even in the presence of aneuploidy, such as trisomy 18, choroid plexus cysts usually resolve.

- Baun J: *Ob/Gyn Sonography: An Illustrated Review*. Pasadena, CA, Davies Publishing, 2016, p 131.
- Gill KA: Fetal syndromes. In Gill KA: *Ultrasound in Obstetrics and Gynecology: A Practitioner's Guide*. Pasadena, CA, Davies Publishing, 2014, p 351.

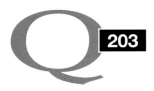

405

Doppler waveforms obtained from an artery supplying an intracranial arteriovenous malformation will exhibit:

a. absent diastolic flow
b. a low pulsatility index
c. decreased velocities
d. triphasic flow

Obstetrics / Fetal Abnormalities

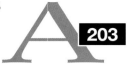

B. A low pulsatility index.

An artery that feeds an arteriovenous malformation will show increased velocities in both systole and diastole. The diastolic velocity especially will be increased, resulting in a waveform demonstrating very low resistance. A waveform that exhibits low resistance will have a low pulsatility index and a low resistivity index.

▶ Rumwell C, McPharlin M: *Vascular Technology: An Illustrated Review*, 5th edition. Pasadena, Davies Publishing, 2015, pp 246–247.

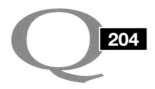

This image demonstrates:

a. alobar holoprosencephaly
b. lobar holoprosencephaly
c. Dandy-Walker malformation
d. hydranencephaly

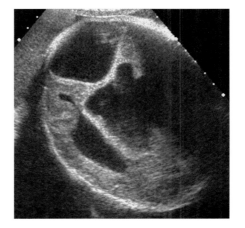

Obstetrics / Fetal Abnormalities

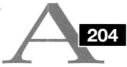

C. Dandy-Walker malformation.

The key findings in this image are the posterior fossa cyst and absent cerebellar vermis. There does appear to be abnormal fluid in the midline, but Dandy-Walker malformation is frequently associated with agenesis of the corpus callosum and enlarged ventricles.

▶ Baun J: *Ob/Gyn Sonography: An Illustrated Review*. Pasadena, CA, Davies Publishing, 2016, p 129.

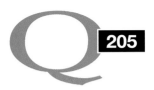

Which of the following is considered a destructive brain process usually caused by hemorrhage?

a. porencephaly
b. holoprosencephaly
c. anencephaly
d. cebocephaly

Obstetrics / Fetal Abnormalities

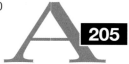

A. Porencephaly.

Porencephaly is destruction of the brain tissue. *Holoprosencephaly* involves midline craniofacial defects. *Anencephaly* is absence of the fetal cranium and most of the brain, and *cebocephaly* is another word for a single-nostril proboscis, seen in holoprosencephaly.

- Baun J: *Ob/Gyn Sonography: An Illustrated Review*. Pasadena, CA, Davies Publishing, 2016, p 134.
- Gill KA: Anomalies associated with polyhydramnios. In Gill KA: *Ultrasound in Obstetrics and Gynecology: A Practitioner's Guide*. Pasadena, CA, Davies Publishing, 2014, p 239.

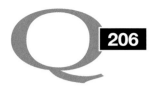

This sonogram of the fetal occiput reveals:

a. omphalocele
b. encephalocele
c. anencephaly
d. iniencephaly

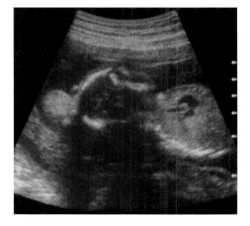

Obstetrics / Fetal Abnormalities

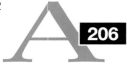

B. Encephalocele.

Encephalocele is herniation of brain tissue and meninges through a bony defect in the calvaria, usually in the occipital region. This axial image demonstrates an occipital encephalocele. The echogenic occipital lobe (O) is herniating into a meningeal sac (H) through a bony calvarial defect (CD).

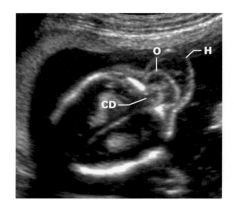

- Baun J: *Ob/Gyn Sonography: An Illustrated Review*. Pasadena, CA, Davies Publishing, 2016, pp 139–140.
- Gill KA: Anomalies associated with polyhydramnios. In Gill KA: *Ultrasound in Obstetrics and Gynecology: A Practitioner's Guide*. Pasadena, CA, Davies Publishing, 2014, pp 232–233.

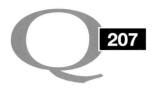

413

This is an image of the fetal head. Additional images demonstrated cyclopia and a proboscis. Collectively the images most likely represent:

a. hydranencephaly
b. hydrocephalus
c. encephalomeningocele
d. holoprosencephaly

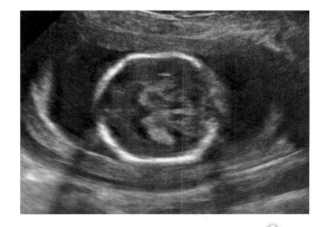

Obstetrics / Fetal Abnormalities

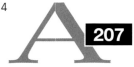

D. Holoprosencephaly.

This image shows absence of the falx cerebri and a common midline ventricle. The alobar form of holoprosencephaly is often associated with severe cleft defects of the face, severe hypotelorism, and proboscis. These findings usually indicate trisomy 13 (Patau syndrome).

- Baun J: *Ob/Gyn Sonography: An Illustrated Review*. Pasadena, CA, Davies Publishing, 2016, pp 126–128.
- Gill KA: Anomalies associated with polyhydramnios. In Gill KA: *Ultrasound in Obstetrics and Gynecology: A Practitioner's Guide*. Pasadena, CA, Davies Publishing, 2014, p 238.

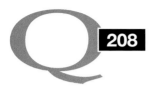

This image demonstrates:

a. Dandy-Walker malformation
b. holoprosencephaly
c. anencephaly
d. ventriculomegaly

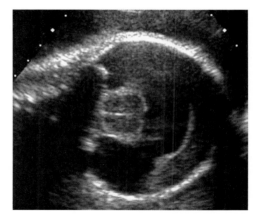

Obstetrics / Fetal Abnormalities

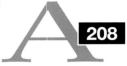

B. Holoprosencephaly.

This image is strongly suggestive of *holoprosencephaly*. There is a large midline monoventricle and fused thalamus with compressed cerebral tissue. *Dandy-Walker* presents with a posterior fossa cyst and absent cerebellar vermis, *anencephaly* is the absence of the cranium and most of the brain, and *ventriculomegaly* is simply dilated ventricles.

▶ Baun J: *Ob/Gyn Sonography: An Illustrated Review*. Pasadena, CA, Davies Publishing, 2016, pp 126–128.

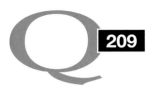

This sonogram of the fetal head depicts:

a. porencephaly
b. choroid plexus cyst
c. hydranencephaly
d. hydrocephalus

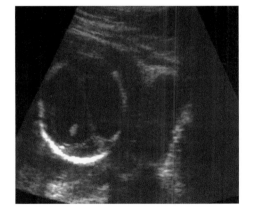

Obstetrics / Fetal Abnormalities

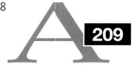

D. Hydrocephalus.

This image shows markedly enlarged lateral ventricles compressing brain tissue, consistent with hydrocephalus. Note that the answer could also be *ventriculomegaly* (not listed as a choice here), which is an enlargement of the ventricles. The term *hydrocephalus* is usually reserved for a case of ventriculomegaly in which the ventricles are under increased pressure. *Porencephaly* is destruction of the parenchymal tissue due to hemorrhage or embolism. *Hydranencephaly* is the complete absence of the cerebral tissue. A choroid plexus cyst does not have this appearance.

- Baun J: *Ob/Gyn Sonography: An Illustrated Review*. Pasadena, CA, Davies Publishing, 2016, pp 122–123.
- Gill KA: *Ultrasound in Obstetrics and Gynecology: A Practitioner's Guide*. Pasadena, CA, Davies Publishing, 2014, pp 232–233.

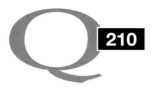

This image demonstrates:

a. hydrocephalus
b. holoprosencephaly
c. hydranencephaly
d. Dandy-Walker malformation

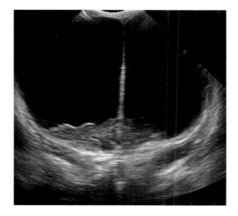

Obstetrics / Fetal Abnormalities

A 210

C. Hydranencephaly.

Hydranencephaly is characterized by complete replacement of cerebral hemispheres by fluid. In hydranencephaly there will be a midline falx, a cerebellum, and a brainstem but no cerebral tissue. With *holoprosencephaly* and *hydrocephalus* there is cerebral tissue, although it may be compressed. In holoprosencephaly the falx will be partially or completely absent. *Dandy-Walker malformation* is a hypoplastic cerebellum and posterior fossa cyst.

▶ Baun J: *Ob/Gyn Sonography: An Illustrated Review*. Pasadena, CA, Davies Publishing, 2016, pp 124–125.

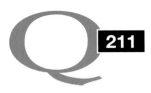

What is the term for a fetal head circumference measuring at least 3 standard deviations below mean for gestational age?

a. microcephaly
b. macrocephaly
c. anencephaly
d. schizencephaly

Obstetrics / Fetal Abnormalities

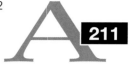

A. Microcephaly.

Microcephaly means "small head," 3 or more standard deviations below normal. *Macrocephaly* is a big head, *anencephaly* is an absent cranium, and *schizencephaly* is a cleft in the brain.

▶ Baun J: *Ob/Gyn Sonography: An Illustrated Review*. Pasadena, CA, Davies Publishing, 2016, p 135.

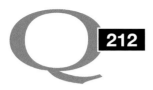

The anomaly seen in this image is most commonly associated with:

a. trisomy 21
b. trisomy 18
c. Beckwith-Wiedemann syndrome
d. holoprosencephaly

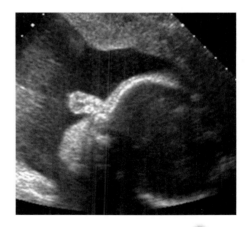

Obstetrics / Fetal Abnormalities

A 212

D. Holoprosencephaly.

The image demonstrates a proboscis, consistent with findings seen in alobar holoprosencephaly. The other syndromes listed do not present with a proboscis. This type of holoprosencephaly may be associated with trisomy 13 (Patau syndrome).

▶ Baun J: *Ob/Gyn Sonography: An Illustrated Review*. Pasadena, CA, Davies Publishing, 2016, pp 126–128.

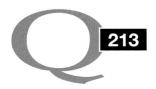

A 27-year-old patient presents for an ultrasound exam with an elevated maternal serum alpha-fetoprotein (MSAFP). What is the finding in this image that correlates with the bloodwork?

a. anencephaly
b. hydranencephaly
c. encephalocele
d. hydrocephalus

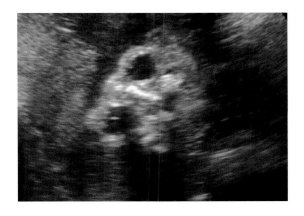

Obstetrics / Fetal Abnormalities / AIT—PACSim

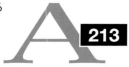

A. Anencephaly.

The MSAFP is elevated in the presence of several conditions, including open neural tube defects and gastroschisis. This image is a coronal section of a fetal face with no discernible skull above the eyes, consistent with anencephaly. With hydranencephaly there is a skull but no cerebrum.

- Baun J: *Ob/Gyn Sonography: An Illustrated Review*. Pasadena, CA, Davies Publishing, 2016, pp 137–138.
- Gill KA: Anomalies associated with polyhydramnios. In Gill KA: *Ultrasound in Obstetrics and Gynecology: A Practitioner's Guide*. Pasadena, CA, Davies Publishing, 2014, p 231.

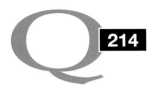

427

A 34-year-old woman presents for an ultrasound exam with elevated maternal serum alpha-fetoprotein (MSAFP). What is the likely cause of the findings in this image?

a. anencephaly
b. omphalocele
c. meningomyelocele
d. hydranencephaly

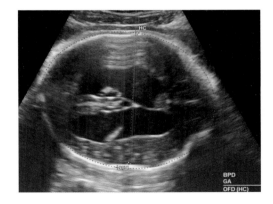

Obstetrics / Fetal Abnormalities / AIT—PACSim

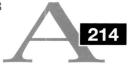

C. Meningomyelocele.

The findings in this image are ventriculomegaly with a dangling choroid plexus and a lemon shape to the frontal bones. These findings can be associated with an open neural tube defect of the spine such as *meningomyelocele* (also called *myelomeningocele*). Not shown in this image is the banana-shaped cerebellum, which is also associated with a meningomyelocele as part of the Arnold-Chiari malformation.

▶ Gill KA: Anomalies associated with polyhydramnios. In Gill KA: *Ultrasound in Obstetrics and Gynecology: A Practitioner's Guide*. Pasadena, CA, Davies Publishing, 2014, pp 233, 234, 240.

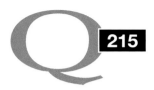

The arrows in this image point to the:

a. mandible
b. soft palate
c. maxilla
d. hard palate

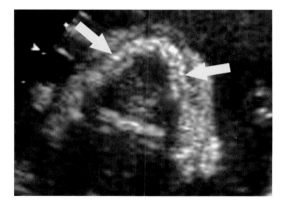

Obstetrics / Fetal Abnormalities / AIT—Hotspot

A 215

C. Maxilla.

The arrows are pointing to the bony maxilla.

▶ Baun J: *Ob/Gyn Sonography: An Illustrated Review*. Pasadena, CA, Davies Publishing, 2016, pp 88, 90–91.

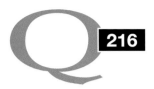

431

Sagittal and axial sections through the fetal orbits presented in this image best demonstrate:

a. anophthalmia
b. hypotelorism
c. hypertelorism
d. cyclopia

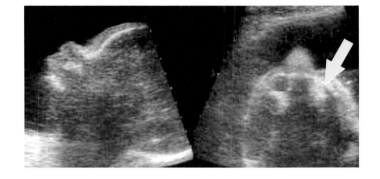

Obstetrics / Fetal Abnormalities

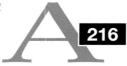

A. Anophthalmia.

Especially visible in the axial image is the absence of an orbit (arrow), termed *anophthalmia*. *Hypotelorism* and *hypertelorism*, respectively, denote orbits that are either too close together or too far apart. *Cyclopia* describes one single, central orbit.

▶ Baun J: *Ob/Gyn Sonography: An Illustrated Review*. Pasadena, CA, Davies Publishing, 2016, pp 100–101.

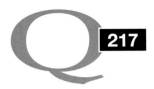

What does this axial section through the fetal face best demonstrate?

a. hypertelorism
b. anophthalmia
c. cyclopia
d. hypotelorism

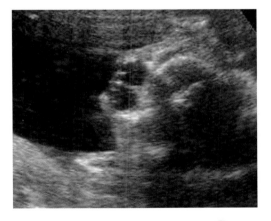

Obstetrics / Fetal Abnormalities

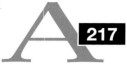

D. Hypotelorism.

This image shows orbits that are too close together, termed *hypotelorism*. *Hypertelorism* refers to orbits that are too far apart, *anophthalmia* is the absence of one or both orbits, and *cyclopia* is a single, central orbit.

▶ Baun J: *Ob/Gyn Sonography: An Illustrated Review*. Pasadena, CA, Davies Publishing, 2016, pp 98–99.

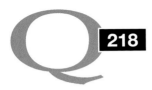

In this image, a midline sagittal sonogram of the fetal face, the arrow points to:

a. cleft palate
b. macroglossia
c. microglossia
d. micrognathia

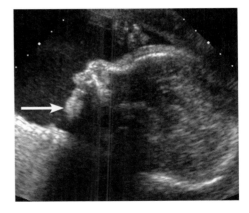

Obstetrics / Fetal Abnormalities / AIT—Hotspot

A 218

D. Micrognathia.

In this image the arrow is pointing to a mandible (chin) that appears too small, a condition termed *micrognathia*. *Macroglossia* and *microglossia* refer to size of the tongue, not visible in this image. Cleft palate is also not demonstrated in this image.

▶ Baun J: *Ob/Gyn Sonography: An Illustrated Review*. Pasadena, CA, Davies Publishing, 2016, pp 101–102.

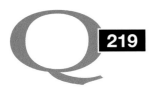

Macroglossia is a common finding in:

a. trisomy 13
b. Beckwith-Wiedemann syndrome
c. maternal phenylketonuria (PKU)
d. Treacher Collins syndrome

Obstetrics / Fetal Abnormalities

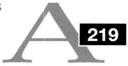

B. Beckwith-Wiedemann syndrome.

Macroglossia is a severely enlarged tongue, which may be associated with Beckwith-Wiedemann syndrome, in which omphalocele, enlargement of intra-abdominal organs, and asymmetry of the fetal limbs may also be observed. Alternatively, macroglossia may be associated with a posterior mass displacing the tongue forward.

- Baun J: *Ob/Gyn Sonography: An Illustrated Review*. Pasadena, CA, Davies Publishing, 2016, pp 102–103.
- Laurenco A, Estroff J: The fetal face and neck. In Rumack CM (ed): *Diagnostic Ultrasound*, 4th edition. St. Louis, Mosby, 2011, pp 1166–1196.

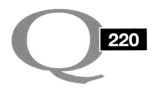

This axial oblique image through the fetal face demonstrates:

a. micrognathia
b. cleft palate
c. macroglossia
d. cleft lip

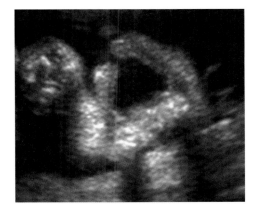

Obstetrics / Fetal Abnormalities

D. Cleft lip.

This image clearly demonstrates a unilateral cleft lip. Although a cleft palate may be present, it is not demonstrated in this image.

▶ Baun J: *Ob/Gyn Sonography: An Illustrated Review*. Pasadena, CA, Davies Publishing, 2016, pp 92–95.

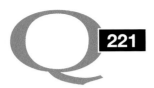

This midline sagittal image through the fetal face best demonstrates:

a. hydrocephalus
b. hypertelorism
c. cyclopia
d. anophthalmia

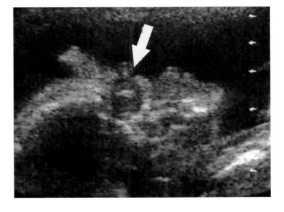

Obstetrics / Fetal Abnormalities

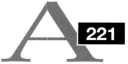

C. Cyclopia.

Normally the orbits are not seen in the midline plane because they are lateral to the midline. In this sagittal image, there is a midline orbit with what appears to be a proboscis superior to the orbit. No other nasal structure is present. This image is consistent with facial characteristics of alobar holoprosencephaly and trisomy 13.

▶ Baun J: *Ob/Gyn Sonography: An Illustrated Review*. Pasadena, CA, Davies Publishing, 2016, pp 99–100.

443

What potential trisomy 21 marker may be measured in the first trimester with or without a nuchal translucency measurement?

a. liver length
b. middle phalanx of the fifth digit
c. nasal bone
d. foot length

Obstetrics / Fetal Abnormalities

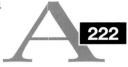

C. Nasal bone.

Hypoplasia of the nasal bone is a potential marker for trisomy 21 (Down syndrome). It may be examined as a routine part of a first trimester ultrasound exam or as part of a first trimester aneuploidy screening protocol. The other fetal parts are not routinely examined in the first trimester.

▶ Baun J: *Ob/Gyn Sonography: An Illustrated Review*. Pasadena, CA, Davies Publishing, 2016, p 82.
▶ Gill KA: *Ultrasound in Obstetrics and Gynecology: A Practitioner's Guide*. Pasadena, CA, Davies Publishing, pp 352–353.

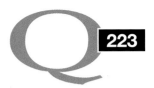

445

The axial section through the fetal head in this image demonstrates:

a. cystic hygroma
b. lymphedema
c. hydrops fetalis
d. teratoma

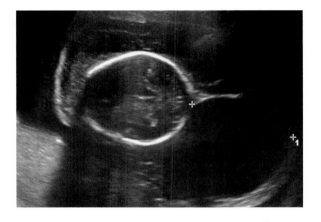

Obstetrics / Fetal Abnormalities

A 223

A. Cystic hygroma.

This image demonstrates large cystic neck tissue, called a *cystic hygroma*. Cystic hygromas may be isolated or may be associated with syndromes such as Turner syndrome.

▶ Baun J: *Ob/Gyn Sonography: An Illustrated Review*. Pasadena, CA, Davies Publishing, 2016, p 105.

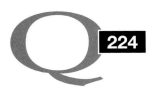 **224**

What is the term for a teratoma that arises from the oral cavity or pharynx?

a. craniopharyngioma
b. epignathus
c. sacral teratoma
d. macroglossia

Obstetrics / Fetal Abnormalities

A **224**

B. Epignathus.

An *epignathus* is an oropharyngeal teratoma that may protrude from the fetal mouth. A *sacral teratoma* occurs at the fetal pelvis. *Macroglossia* is an enlarged fetal tongue. A *craniopharyngioma* is a brain tumor near the pituitary gland.

▶ Baun J: *Ob/Gyn Sonography: An Illustrated Review*. Pasadena, CA, Davies Publishing, 2016, p 104.

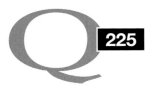

The arrow in this sagittal section through the fetal neck is pointing to a:

a. teratoma
b. cystic hygroma
c. multinodular goiter
d. lymphoma

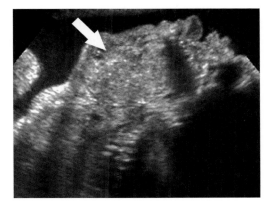

Obstetrics / Fetal Abnormalities / AIT—Hotspot

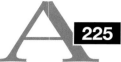

A. Teratoma.

The most likely pathology of the choices listed is teratoma. This image demonstrates a fetal neck mass (arrow) that appears to be extending the head abnormally. The hyperextension of the fetal neck from the mass may obstruct fetal swallowing, causing polyhydramnios. Cystic hygromas arise from the back of the neck and are cystic with septations, not solid like this mass.

▶ Baun J: *Ob/Gyn Sonography: An Illustrated Review*. Pasadena, CA, Davies Publishing, 2016, pp 103–104.

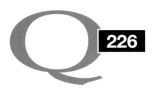

The coronal section through the fetal neck presented in this image best demonstrates:

a. cystic hygroma
b. teratoma
c. increased nuchal translucency
d. thyroglossal duct cysts

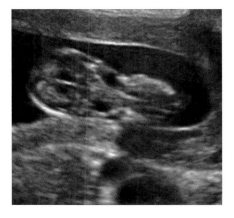

Obstetrics / Fetal Abnormalities

A 226

D. Thyroglossal duct cysts.

This coronal image demonstrates fluid in the neck, consistent with thyroglossal duct cysts. The *thyroglossal duct* is the embryologic tract that the thyroid uses to reach its normal location at the base of the neck. Sometimes cysts form within this tract. A *cystic hygroma* would be demonstrated as fluid in the axial plane around the neck, and a *teratoma* is a heterogeneous mass. An increased *nuchal translucency* would best be seen in the sagittal plane.

▶ Baun J: *Ob/Gyn Sonography: An Illustrated Review*. Pasadena, CA, Davies Publishing, 2016, p 103.

Cystic hygroma is most commonly found in association with which of the following abnormal congenital chromosomal conditions?

a. trisomy 13
b. trisomy 21
c. Treacher Collins syndrome
d. Turner syndrome

Obstetrics / Fetal Abnormalities

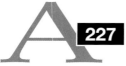

D. Turner syndrome.

Turner syndrome is characterized by an abnormal karyotype, 45,X. Only a single sex chromosome, an X chromosome, is present, and affected fetuses are therefore considered female. Turner syndrome may present in utero as a cystic hygroma. Babies born with Turner syndrome characteristically have a webbed neck and nonfunctioning, streak ovaries. None of the other choices listed commonly presents with a cystic hygroma.

▶ Baun J: *Ob/Gyn Sonography: An Illustrated Review*. Pasadena, CA, Davies Publishing, 2016, p 106.

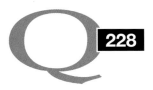

The finding in this image suggests:

a. Arnold-Chiari malformation
b. Dandy-Walker malformation
c. limb–body wall complex
d. congenital pulmonary airway malformation (CPAM)

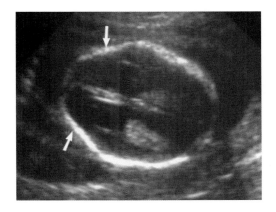

Obstetrics / Fetal Abnormalities

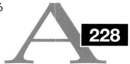

A. Arnold-Chiari malformation.

Findings consistent with Arnold-Chiari malformation include open neural tube defects of the spine, such as spina bifida aperta. In Arnold-Chiari, there are pointed frontal bones (arrows), which result in an appearance called the "lemon sign" seen in this image. There may also be hydrocephalus, an obliterated cisterna magna, and a cerebellum inferiorly displaced into the foramen magnum.

▶ Baun J: *Ob/Gyn Sonography: An Illustrated Review*. Pasadena, CA, Davies Publishing, 2016, pp 142–143.
▶ Gill KA: Anomalies associated with polyhydramnios. In Gill KA: *Ultrasound in Obstetrics and Gynecology: A Practitioner's Guide*. Pasadena, CA, Davies Publishing, 2014, p 234.

The sonogram of this fetal profile reveals:

a. encephalocele
b. anencephaly
c. iniencephaly
d. meningomyelocele

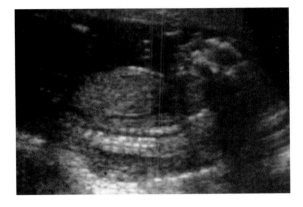

Obstetrics / Fetal Abnormalities

457

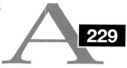

B. Anencephaly.

Anencephaly is an absence of the cranial vault and brain tissue. It is a lethal neural tube defect. In this sagittal image there are two linear echogenic structures in the region of the fetal head, with the most inferior representing the upper jaw and the most superior representing the orbits. No cranium is seen superior to the orbits, indicating anencephaly.

▶ Baun J: *Ob/Gyn Sonography: An Illustrated Review*. Pasadena, CA, Davies Publishing, 2016, pp 137–138.

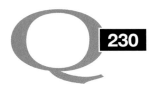

The arrow and cursors in this image are delineating a:

a. cystic teratoma
b. cystic hygroma
c. branchial cleft cyst
d. meningomyelocele

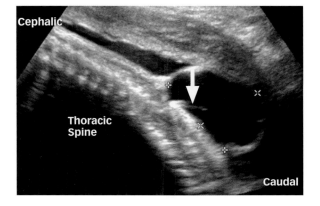

Obstetrics / Fetal Abnormalities / AIT—Hotspot

A 230

D. Meningomyelocele.

This sagittal image of the spine is demonstrating a meningomyelocele, an open neural tube defect of the spine. In a *meningocele*, only the meninges and cerebrospinal fluid (CSF) are in the defect. In a *meningomyelocele*, CSF, meninges, and spinal cord are present in the defect.

▶ Baun J: *Ob/Gyn Sonography: An Illustrated Review*. Pasadena, CA, Davies Publishing, 2016, p 142.

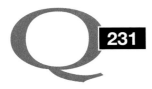

This image demonstrates:

a. spina bifida
b. Dandy-Walker malformation
c. cranial dysostosis
d. anencephaly

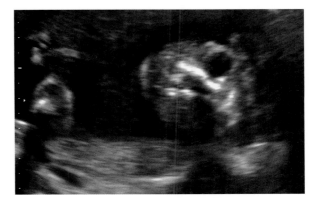

Obstetrics / Fetal Abnormalities

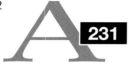

D. Anencephaly.

This is a coronal image of a fetus with anencephaly. Note, superior to the orbits, the absence of a cranium.

▶ Baun J: *Ob/Gyn Sonography: An Illustrated Review*. Pasadena, CA, Davies Publishing, 2016, pp 137–138.

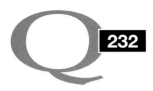

Effacement of the cerebellar hemispheres in a fetus with spina bifida creates a sonographic finding known as the:

a. lemon sign
b. banana sign
c. strawberry sign
d. pear sign

Obstetrics / Fetal Abnormalities

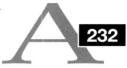

B. Banana sign.

The "banana sign" is the sonographic appearance of a compression of the cerebellum that obliterates the region of the cisterna magna and distorts the head shape.

- Baun J: *Ob/Gyn Sonography: An Illustrated Review*. Pasadena, CA, Davies Publishing, 2016, pp 142–143.
- Sauerbrei EE: The fetal spine. In Rumack CM (ed): *Diagnostic Ultrasound*, 4th edition. St. Louis, Mosby, 2011, pp 1245–1272.

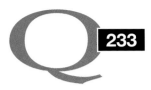

What is the name of the condition in which the spine is open for the majority of its length?

a. rachischisis
b. scoliosis
c. kyphosis
d. platyspondylisis

Obstetrics / Fetal Abnormalities

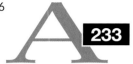

A. Rachischisis.

Rachischisis (also referred to as *myeloschisis*) is a severe spinal defect that extends throughout most of the spine. *Scoliosis* is lateral curvature of spine, *kyphosis* is a curvature that causes a so-called hump, and *platyspondylisis* (also called *platyspondyly*) is a flattening or widening of the vertebral bodies.

- Baun J: *Ob/Gyn Sonography: An Illustrated Review*. Pasadena, CA, Davies Publishing, 2016, pp 141, 142.
- Gill KA: Anomalies associated with polyhydramnios. In Gill KA: *Ultrasound in Obstetrics and Gynecology: A Practitioner's Guide*. Pasadena, CA, Davies Publishing, 2014, p 240.

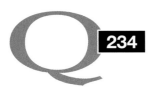

Which of these forms of spina bifida is typically diagnosed postnatally?

a. aperta
b. occulta
c. dysraphism
d. lumbosacral

Obstetrics / Fetal Abnormalities

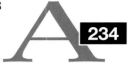

B. Occulta.

Spina bifida occulta is the milder form of spina bifida, consisting of a defect in the posterior bony neural arch that remains "hidden" by intact overlying musculature, fascia, and skin. It is rarely demonstrated sonographically in the fetus. *Spinal dysraphism* is another term for spina bifida, *aperta* is a different form of spina bifida, and *lumbosacral* refers to a location on the spine.

▶ Baun J: *Ob/Gyn Sonography: An Illustrated Review*. Pasadena, CA, Davies Publishing, 2016, p 141.

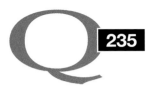

An open defect along the posterior spine with protrusion of neural tissue and meninges is called:

a. spina bifida occulta
b. spina bifida aperta
c. iniencephaly
d. encephalocele

Obstetrics / Fetal Abnormalities

235

B. Spina bifida aperta.

The term *spina bifida* is nonspecifc and may be broken down into open defects, called *spina bifida aperta*, and closed defects, called *spina bifida occulta*. Spina bifida aperta can be separated into meningocele, in which only meninges and cerebrospinal fluid (CSF) protrude, and myelomeningocele (also called meningomyelocele), in which spinal cord, meninges, and CSF protrude. *Iniencephaly* is a spinal defect of the cervicothoracic spine, and *encephalocele* is protrusion of intracranial contents through a bony skull defect.

▶ Baun J: *Ob/Gyn Sonography: An Illustrated Review*. Pasadena, CA, Davies Publishing, 2016, p 142.

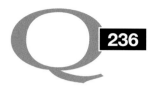

This patient presented with elevated alpha-fetoprotein (AFP) and was referred for sonographic evaluation. These images show:

a. spina bifida occulta
b. spina bifida with meningocele
c. spina bifida with myelomeningocele
d. rachischisis

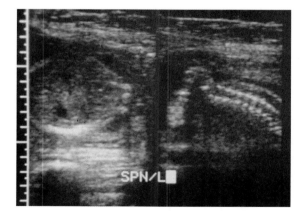

Obstetrics / Fetal Abnormalities / AIT—PACSim

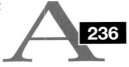

A 236

C. Spina bifida with myelomeningocele.

Spina bifida occulta would not present with a mass and is usually difficult to see sonographically. A meningocele would be cystic. In rachischisis the spine is open throughout its length and the spinal cord is exposed.

- Baun J: *Ob/Gyn Sonography: An Illustrated Review*. Pasadena, CA, Davies Publishing, 2016, p 142.
- Gill KA: Anomalies associated with polyhydramnios. In Gill KA: *Ultrasound in Obstetrics and Gynecology: A Practitioner's Guide*. Pasadena, CA, Davies Publishing, 2014, pp 240–241.

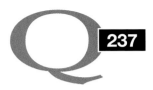

Visualization of a fetus in the "stargazer" posture is suspicious for:

a. anencephaly
b. iniencephaly
c. spina bifida
d. encephalocele

Obstetrics / Fetal Abnormalities

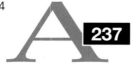

B. Iniencephaly.

The so-called stargazer position describes the extreme extension of the fetal neck and head seen with iniencephaly. This fetal position does not occur with the other anomalies listed.

▶ Baun J: *Ob/Gyn Sonography: An Illustrated Review*. Pasadena, CA, Davies Publishing, 2016, p 140.

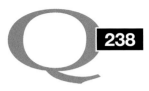

This image demonstrates:

a. encephalocele
b. neck teratoma
c. cystic hygroma
d. nuchal fold thickening

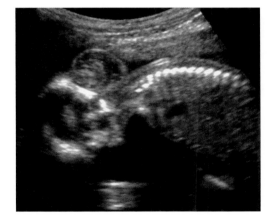

Obstetrics / Fetal Abnormalities

A **238**

A. Encephalocele.

This image is that of a posterior encephalocele. Teratomas can have a similar appearance but are usually not in this location and are uncommon compared to encephaloceles. Cystic hygroma is fluid around the fetal neck, and this is not a typical appearance for a thickened nuchal fold.

▶ Baun J: *Ob/Gyn Sonography: An Illustrated Review*. Pasadena, CA, Davies Publishing, 2016, pp 139–140.

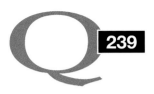

By which menstrual week does physiologic herniation of the fetal midgut usually resolve?

a. 6
b. 8
c. 12
d. 10

Obstetrics / Fetal Abnormalities

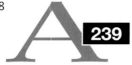

C. 12.

Prior to 12 weeks, herniation of the intestines into the base of the umbilical cord is normal because of rapid organ growth. This herniation should not be visible after 12 weeks' menstrual age.

▶ Baun J: *Ob/Gyn Sonography: An Illustrated Review*. Pasadena, CA, Davies Publishing, 2016, pp 220–221.
▶ Sliman MH, Gill KA: The first trimester. In Gill KA: *Ultrasound in Obstetrics and Gynecology: A Practitioner's Guide*. Pasadena, CA, Davies Publishing, 2014, p 100.

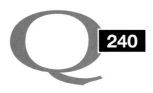

479

What is the name of an anterior abdominal midline mass at the level of the cord insertion and covered with a membrane?

a. gastroschisis
b. cloacal exstrophy
c. omphalocele
d. limb–body wall complex

Obstetrics / Fetal Abnormalities

C. Omphalocele.

Omphalocele is a ventral wall defect covered by skin and may contain fetal bowel and/or organs such as the liver. Omphalocele is commonly associated with chromosomal defects and syndromes.

▶ Abbott JF: The fetal abdominal wall and gastrointestinal tract. In Rumack CM (ed): *Diagnostic Ultrasound*, 4th edition. St. Louis, Mosby, 2011, pp 1327–1352.

▶ Baun J: *Ob/Gyn Sonography: An Illustrated Review*. Pasadena, CA, Davies Publishing, 2016, p 226.

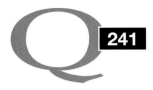

The echogenic area adjacent to the fetal abdomen in this image represents:

a. omphalocele
b. tangled umbilical cord
c. gastroschisis
d. fetal extremities

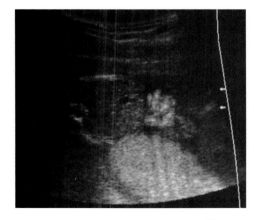

Obstetrics / Fetal Abnormalities

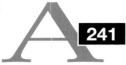

C. Gastroschisis.

Gastroschisis is a paraumbilical defect in the abdominal wall through which fetal bowel herniates into the amniotic cavity, as demonstrated in the transverse image of the fetal abdomen at the level of the abdominal cord insertion site. It usually herniates to the right of the umbilical cord insertion. Gastroschisis is not typically associated with chromosomal anomalies and can be surgically repaired.

▶ Baun J: *Ob/Gyn Sonography: An Illustrated Review*. Pasadena, CA, Davies Publishing, 2016, pp 227–228.
▶ Gill KA: Anomalies associated with polyhydramnios. In Gill KA: *Ultrasound in Obstetrics and Gynecology: A Practitioner's Guide*. Pasadena, CA, Davies Publishing, 2014, pp 253–254.

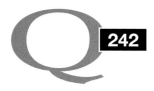

483

Based on this image, which of the following choices would be the most likely diagnosis?

a. gastroschisis
b. extralobar sequestration
c. prune belly syndrome
d. extracorporeal liver

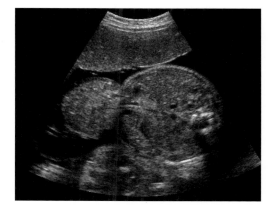

Obstetrics / Fetal Abnormalities

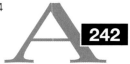

D. Extracorporeal liver.

This transverse image of the fetal abodmen at the level of the abdominal cord insertion site demontrates a soft-tissue organ, most likely liver, outside of the abdomen. With *gastroschisis*, the herniated fetal bowel is free-floating in the amniotic fluid. *Extralobar sequestration* involves an accessory lung lobe. *Prune belly syndrome* involves severe distention of the urinary bladder.

▸ Baun J: *Ob/Gyn Sonography: An Illustrated Review*. Pasadena, CA, Davies Publishing, 2016, p 228.
▸ Gill KA: Anomalies associated with polyhydramnios. In Gill KA: *Ultrasound in Obstetrics and Gynecology: A Practitioner's Guide*. Pasadena, CA, Davies Publishing, 2014, p 255.

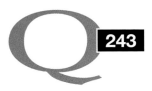

What is the name for a uniformly lethal congenital abdominal wall defect characterized by absent umbilical cord and exteriorization of abdominal contents that attach directly to the placental surface?

a. gastroschisis
b. limb–body wall complex
c. cloacal exstrophy
d. abdominoschisis

Obstetrics / Fetal Abnormalities

A **243**

B. Limb–body wall complex.

Limb–body wall complex is a severe, lethal abnormality in which the ventral wall is attached to the placenta and the organs are exteriorized.

▶ Baun J: *Ob/Gyn Sonography: An Illustrated Review*. Pasadena, CA, Davies Publishing, 2016, pp 229–230.

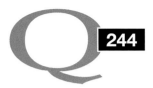

The sonographic findings seen in this image of the fetal pelvis are most consistent with:

a. bladder exstrophy
b. diaphragmatic hernia
c. duodenal atresia
d. sacrococcygeal teratoma

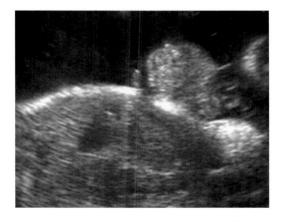

Obstetrics / Fetal Abnormalities

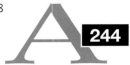

A. Bladder exstrophy.

This image is that of a long-axis fetal pelvis with an anterior soft-tissue mass. The fetal bladder is not visualized. Given the choices listed, the most likely explanation is bladder exstrophy. *Bladder exstrophy* is a ventral wall defect characterized by exteriorization of the bladder. The urinary bladder is *everted* (turned "inside out") so no bladder will be visualized.

▶ Baun J: *Ob/Gyn Sonography: An Illustrated Review*. Pasadena, CA, Davies Publishing, 2016, p 231.
▶ Gill KA: Anomalies associated with polyhydramnios. In Gill KA: *Ultrasound in Obstetrics and Gynecology: A Practitioner's Guide*. Pasadena, CA, Davies Publishing, 2014, p 255.

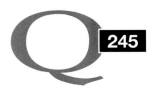

Q 245

Which of the following would cause elevated levels of maternal serum alpha-fetoprotein (MSAFP)?

a. gastroschisis
b. omphalocele
c. congenital diaphragmatic hernia
d. umbilical vein varix

Obstetrics / Fetal Abnormalities

A **245**

A. Gastroschisis.

Gastroschisis is a protrusion of the fetal bowel through an open ventral wall defect, adjacent to the umbilical cord. This defect is not covered by skin, as with an omphalocele, so intra-abdominal contents are open to the amniotic fluid. Therefore, the MSAFP will be elevated.

▶ Baun J: *Ob/Gyn Sonography: An Illustrated Review*. Pasadena, CA, Davies Publishing, 2016, p 273.

▶ Gill KA: Introduction to diagnostic ultrasound. In Gill KA: *Ultrasound in Obstetrics and Gynecology: A Practitioner's Guide*. Pasadena, CA, Davies Publishing, 2014, p 253.

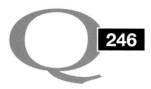

This image best demonstrates:

a. duodenal atresia
b. ectopia cordis
c. congenital pulmonary airway malformation (CPAM)
d. diaphragmatic hernia

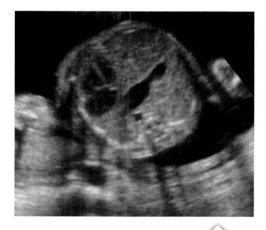

Obstetrics / Fetal Abnormalities

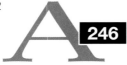

D. Diaphragmatic hernia.

In this image the fetal stomach is at the level of the fetal heart, indicating a *diaphragmatic hernia*. Not only are the two structures at the same level, but the fetal heart is being displaced as well. *Duodenal atresia* presents as a "double bubble" sign in the abdomen, *ectopia cordis* presents as the heart protruding through a thoracic wall defect, and *CPAM* most typically presents as an echogenic mass in the fetal chest.

▶ Baun J: *Ob/Gyn Sonography: An Illustrated Review*. Pasadena, CA, Davies Publishing, 2016, pp 168–169.

247

A congenital abnormality of lung development characterized by the replacement of normal tissue with nonfunctioning cystic tissue is called:

a. diaphragmatic hernia
b. congenital pulmonary airway malformation (CPAM)
c. pulmonary sequestration
d. pulmonary hypoplasia

Obstetrics / Fetal Abnormalities

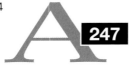

B. Congenital pulmonary airway malformation (CPAM).

CPAM (also known as *CCAM, congenital cystic adenomatoid malformation,* or *CAML, cystic adenomatoid malformation of the lung*) is a benign fetal lung mass that receives its arterial supply from the pulmonary arterial branches. The lesion may be large and macrocystic (type 1); it may consist of multiple small cysts (type 2); or it may be microcystic, appearing as an echogenic mass because the cysts are so small (type 3). Type 1 is the most common type of CPAM. *Pulmonary sequestration* is an extra lobe of lung and appears as a solid mass.

▶ Baun J: *Ob/Gyn Sonography: An Illustrated Review*. Pasadena, CA, Davies Publishing, 2016, p 170.

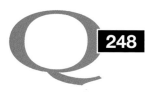

An accessory fragment of lung with a separate systemic arterial circulation and with no connection to the tracheobronchial tree is known as:

a. congenital pulmonary airway malformation
b. diaphragmatic hernia
c. pulmonary sequestration
d. diaphragmatic eventration

Obstetrics / Fetal Abnormalities

A 248

C. Pulmonary sequestration.

Pulmonary sequestration appears as an echogenic mass most commonly above the diaphragm, although it can occur below the diaphragm. This lesion connects to the aorta for its arterial blood supply.

▶ Baun J: *Ob/Gyn Sonography: An Illustrated Review*. Pasadena, CA, Davies Publishing, 2016, pp 167–168.

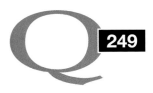

The sonographic appearance of pulmonary sequestration can be similar to that of:

a. complete common atrioventricular canal
b. congenital cystic adenomatoid malformation of the lung
c. anomalous insertion of the pulmonary veins
d. congenital diaphragmatic hernia

Obstetrics / Fetal Abnormalities

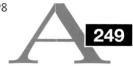

B. Congenital cystic adenomatoid malformation of the lung.

Both pulmonary sequestration and the microcystic type of *congenital cystic adenomatoid malformation of the lung* (CCAM type 3)—also known as *congenital pulmonary airway malformation* (CPAM) or *congenital cystic adenomatoid malformation* (CCAM)—appear as hyperechoic masses adjacent to or within the lung and may cause displacement of the heart.

▶ Baun J: *Ob/Gyn Sonography: An Illustrated Review*. Pasadena, CA, Davies Publishing, 2016, pp 167–168, 170.
▶ Gill KA: Anomalies associated with polyhydramnios. In Gill KA: *Ultrasound in Obstetrics and Gynecology: A Practitioner's Guide*. Pasadena, CA, Davies Publishing, 2014, pp 245–246.

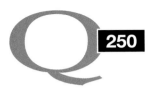

499

The arrow in this image points to:

a. pulmonary sequestration
b. pleural effusion
c. pericardial tumor
d. congenital pulmonary airway malformation

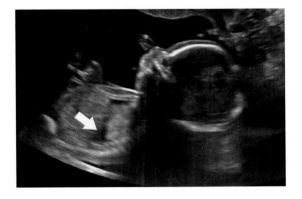

Obstetrics / Fetal Abnormalities / AIT—Hotspot

B. Pleural effusion.

The arrow in this image points to fluid in the fetal thorax consistent with pleural effusion.

Baun J: *Ob/Gyn Sonography: An Illustrated Review*. Pasadena, CA, Davies Publishing, 2016, pp 166–167.

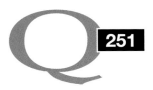

Q 251

What does this image demonstrate?

a. normal lung/liver echogenicity
b. pulmonary sequestration
c. congenital pulmonary airway malformation
d. cystic fibrosis

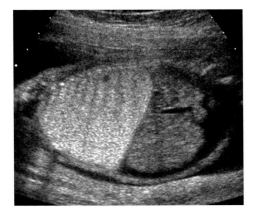

Obstetrics / Fetal Abnormalities

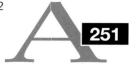

C. Congenital pulmonary airway malformation.

Congenital pulmonary airway malformation (*CPAM*, also known as *CCAM, congenital cystic adenomatoid malformation,* or *CAML, cystic adenomatoid malformation of the lung*) is abnormal lung tissue presenting as a mass. There are different types (see the answer to question 247). Pictured here is the type 3 (microcystic) type.

▶ Baun J: *Ob/Gyn Sonography: An Illustrated Review*. Pasadena, CA, Davies Publishing, 2016, p 170.

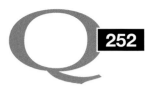

Bladder exstrophy is caused by a defect in the development of the:

a. paramesonephric müllerian ducts
b. mesonephric (wolffian) duct
c. ureteric buds
d. cloacal membrane

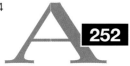

D. Cloacal membrane.

Bladder exstrophy is a defect in the cloacal membrane causing an everted bladder that is exposed to the amniotic cavity. It can be differentiated from omphalocele because of its location inferior to the umbilical cord insertion site.

- Baun J: *Ob/Gyn Sonography: An Illustrated Review*. Pasadena, CA, Davies Publishing, 2016, pp 230–231.
- Fong KW, Robertson JE, Maxwell CV: The fetal urogenital tract. In Rumack CM (ed): *Diagnostic Ultrasound*, 4th edition. St. Louis, Mosby, 2011, pp 1353–1388.

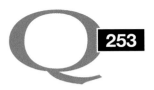

253

Your patient presents with a history of chronic absence of amniotic fluid in a severely oligohydramniotic sac. What is the term for the structural and developmental fetal abnormalities associated with this condition?

a. Potter sequence
b. bilateral renal agenesis
c. Beckwith-Wiedemann syndrome
d. Zellweger syndrome

Obstetrics / Fetal Abnormalities

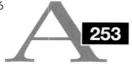

A. Potter sequence.

Potter sequence is a collection of findings that are present in the setting of severe oligohydramnios or anhydramnios. Any syndrome or congenital anomaly that causes a severe lack of amniotic fluid may lead to Potter sequence, presenting as flattened fetal facies and limb anomalies such as clubfoot and abnormally contracted joints. *Pulmonary hypoplasia*, a potentially fatal condition, and *intrauterine growth restriction* (IUGR) are often associated with Potter sequence.

▶ Baun J: *Ob/Gyn Sonography: An Illustrated Review*. Pasadena, CA, Davies Publishing, 2016, pp 253–258.

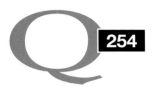

The presence of a kidney outside its expected position in the renal fossa is called:

a. ectopic ureterocele
b. renal ectopia
c. renal agenesis
d. renal dysplasia

Obstetrics / Fetal Abnormalities

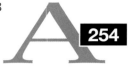

B. Renal ectopia.

Renal ectopia is a kidney not located in its usual position in the renal fossa. The most common location for an ectopic kidney is in the pelvis.

▶ Baun J: *Ob/Gyn Sonography: An Illustrated Review*. Pasadena, CA, Davies Publishing, 2016, pp 252–253.

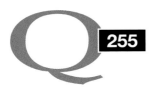

In most fetuses with bilateral renal agenesis, postnatal mortality results from:

a. clubfoot
b. polyhydramnios
c. pulmonary hypoplasia
d. limb contractures

A 255

C. Pulmonary hypoplasia.

Pulmonary hypoplasia is the result of oligohydramnios that does not allow the fetal lungs to expand with fluid and develop, leading to death. Pulmonary hypoplasia may be caused by renal agenesis, congenital diaphragmatic hernia, and conditions that lead to a small fetal thorax such as some skeletal dysplasias. The other choices listed are nonfatal sequelae of severe oligohydramnios.

▶ Baun J: *Ob/Gyn Sonography: An Illustrated Review*. Pasadena, CA, Davies Publishing, 2016, p 252.

▶ Fong KW, Robertson JE, Maxwell CV: The fetal urogenital tract. In Rumack CM (ed): *Diagnostic Ultrasound*, 4th edition. St. Louis, Mosby, 2011, pp 1353–1388.

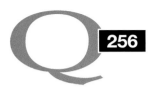

511

The findings seen in this image are most consistent with:

a. ureteropelvic junction obstruction
b. ectopic ureterocele
c. primary megaureter
d. posterior urethral valves

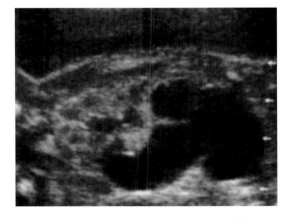

Obstetrics / Fetal Abnormalities

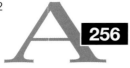

A. Ureteropelvic junction obstruction.

The image shows a kidney with a ureteropelvic junction (UPJ) obstruction in the upper pole. This kidney probably has a duplicated collecting system. Obstruction most commonly occurs in the upper pole of a duplicated collecting system.

▶ Baun J: *Ob/Gyn Sonography: An Illustrated Review*. Pasadena, CA, Davies Publishing, 2016, pp 259–260.

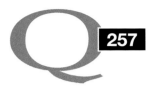

The sonographic findings seen in this image are most consistent with:

a. polycystic kidney disease
b. hydronephrosis
c. ureteropelvic junction obstruction
d. multicystic dysplastic kidney disease

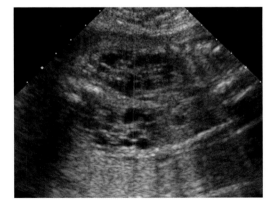

Obstetrics / Fetal Abnormalities

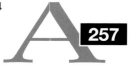

D. Multicystic dysplastic kidney disease.

Multicystic dysplastic kidney disease (MCDKD) is characterized by cysts forming in the kidneys. The condition is usually unilateral, which is fortunate as the affected kidney is typically nonfunctioning. The contralateral kidney must be examined for pathology. When the condition is bilateral, as seen in this fetus, MCDKD is usually fatal.

▶ Baun J: *Ob/Gyn Sonography: An Illustrated Review*. Pasadena, CA, Davies Publishing, 2016, pp 255–256.

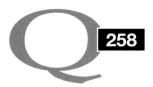

The sonographic findings seen in this image are most consistent with:

a. posterior urethral valves
b. prune belly syndrome
c. ectopic ureterocele
d. primary megacystis

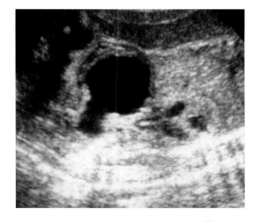

Obstetrics / Fetal Abnormalities

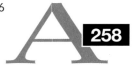

A. Posterior urethral valves.

This image demonstrates the classic keyhole-shaped defect seen in posterior urethral valves (PUV). This condition occurs only in males and is an obstruction of the urethra that causes massive bladder dilatation, hydroureter, and hydronephrosis. Severe oligohydramnios develops as a result of the obstruction.

▶ Baun J: *Ob/Gyn Sonography: An Illustrated Review*. Pasadena, CA, Davies Publishing, 2016, pp 262–263.

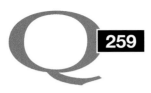

The absence of one or both fetal kidneys is called:

a. renal aplasia
b. renal dysplasia
c. renal ectopia
d. renal agenesis

Obstetrics / Fetal Abnormalities

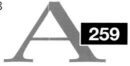

D. Renal agenesis.

Renal agenesis means absence of one or both kidneys (or the failure of the kidneys to develop). When the condition is bilateral, it is uniformly fatal. It is important always to document two fetal kidneys as part of a fetal anatomic survey.

▶ Baun J: *Ob/Gyn Sonography: An Illustrated Review*. Pasadena, CA, Davies Publishing, 2016, pp 251–252.

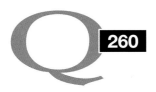

The sonographic findings seen in this image are most consistent with:

a. multicystic dysplastic kidney
b. polycystic kidney disease
c. intestinal atresia
d. hydronephrosis

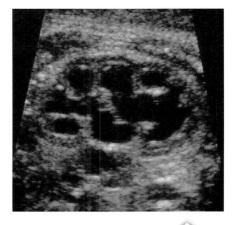

Obstetrics / Fetal Abnormalities

A 260

D. Hydronephrosis.

This is an image of a kidney with dilated calyces, or *caliectasis*, consistent with hydronephrosis. The dilated calyces look different from frank cysts, as would be seen in multicystic dysplastic kidney disease or autosomal dominant polycystic kidney disease.

▶ Baun J: *Ob/Gyn Sonography: An Illustrated Review*. Pasadena, CA, Davies Publishing, 2016, pp 258–259.

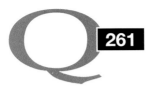

Q 261

These images demonstrate fetal kidneys. What is the most likely diagnosis?

a. autosomal recessive polycystic kidneys
b. normal kidneys
c. multicystic dysplastic kidneys
d. hydronephrotic kidneys

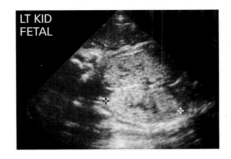

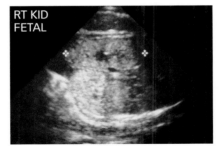

Obstetrics / Fetal Abnormalities

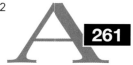

A. Autosomal recessive polycystic kidneys.

Normal kidneys show a hyperechoic center and hypoechoic cortex, while multicystic and hydronephrotic kidneys are more cystic in appearance. *Autosomal recessive* (formerly called *infantile*) *polycystic kidneys* are enlarged and markedly echogenic. The preferred terminology for this condition is *autosomal recessive polycystic kidney disease.*

- Baun J: *Ob/Gyn Sonography: An Illustrated Review*. Pasadena, CA, Davies Publishing, 2016, pp 253–254.
- Niudet P: Autosomal recessive polycystic kidney disease in children. UpToDate. Available at https://www-uptodate-com.proxy1.lib.tju.edu/contents/autosomal-recessive-polycystic-kidney-disease-in-children?source=machineLearning&search=autosomal+recessive+polycystic+kidney+disease&selectedTitle=1%7E25&sectionRank=1&anchor=H4#H4.
- Rodriguez J, Gill KA: Anomalies associated with oligohydramnios. In Gill KA: *Ultrasound in Obstetrics and Gynecology: A Practitioner's Guide*. Pasadena, CA, Davies Publishing, 2014, pp 274–275.

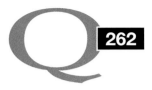

Bilateral fetal hydronephrosis usually means:

a. There is an obstruction at the ureteropelvic junction.
b. There is an obstruction along one of the ureters.
c. There is an obstruction at the urethral outflow tract.
d. There is polyhydramnios.

Obstetrics / Fetal Abnormalities

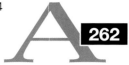 **262**

C. There is an obstruction at the urethral outflow tract.

When the entire urinary tract is obstructed, the source is usually posterior urethral valves or other bladder outlet obstruction. Ureteropelvic junction obstructions affect the kidneys only, not the ureters and bladder. The prognosis for bilateral obstruction depends on when the process develops and whether intervention can be performed to salvage at least one kidney and allow for enough amniotic fluid production so that the lungs can develop properly.

▶ Baun J: *Ob/Gyn Sonography: An Illustrated Review*. Pasadena, CA, Davies Publishing, 2016, pp 258–262.
▶ Rodriguez J, Gill KA: Anomalies associated with oligohydramnios. In Gill KA: *Ultrasound in Obstetrics and Gynecology: A Practitioner's Guide*. Pasadena, CA, Davies Publishing, 2014, pp 276–277.

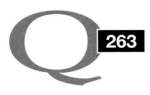

Multicystic dysplastic kidneys are usually:

a. unilateral and nonfunctional
b. bilateral but functional
c. bilateral and nonfunctional
d. unilateral but functional

Obstetrics / Fetal Abnormalities

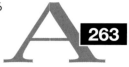

A. Unilateral and nonfunctional.

Although the multicystic kidney does not function well if at all, the condition is typically unilateral; therefore the opposite kidney compensates for the loss of function on the multicystic side. When multicystic dysplasia is bilateral, usually one kidney is affected more than the other, with some function present.

- Baun J: *Ob/Gyn Sonography: An Illustrated Review*. Pasadena, CA, Davies Publishing, 2016, pp 255–256.
- Rodriguez J, Gill KA: Anomalies associated with oligohydramnios. In Gill KA: *Ultrasound in Obstetrics and Gynecology: A Practitioner's Guide*. Pasadena, CA, Davies Publishing, 2014, p 276.

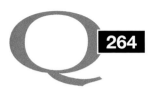

If one fetal kidney shows dilatation of the fetal renal pelvis and calyces but there is no evidence of a dilated ureter or bladder, the most likely diagnosis would be:

a. obstruction at the ureterovesical junction (UVJ)
b. obstruction at the ureteropelvic junction (UPJ)
c. posterior urethral valves (PUV)
d. renal hypoplasia

Obstetrics / Fetal Abnormalities

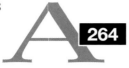

B. Obstruction at the ureteropelvic junction (UPJ).

A UVJ and mid-ureteral junction would show hydronephrosis and dilated ureter, usually unilateral. PUV would show dilatation of the entire urinary tract, including both kidneys, the ureters, and the bladder.

- Baun J: *Ob/Gyn Sonography: An Illustrated Review*. Pasadena, CA, Davies Publishing, 2016, pp 259–260.
- Rodriguez J, Gill KA: Anomalies associated with oligohydramnios. In Gill KA: *Ultrasound in Obstetrics and Gynecology: A Practitioner's Guide*. Pasadena, CA, Davies Publishing, 2014, p 279.

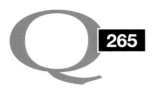

This image demonstrates:

a. normal fetal abdomen
b. bilateral renal agenesis
c. hepatosplenic calcifications
d. echogenic bowel

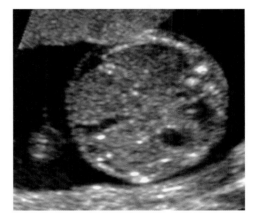

Obstetrics / Fetal Abnormalities

A 265

C. Hepatosplenic calcifications.

Fetal abdominal calcifications are not specific to a disease process and are usually benign. In this image the calcifications are in the liver and spleen and may be benign or related to maternal infections, vascular problems, and/or chromosomal abnormalities.

▶ Baun J: *Ob/Gyn Sonography: An Illustrated Review*. Pasadena, CA, Davies Publishing, 2016, pp 238–239.

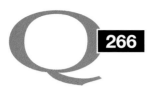

What does this image best demonstrate?

a. duodenal atresia
b. hepatic cysts
c. ovarian cysts
d. meconium peritonitis

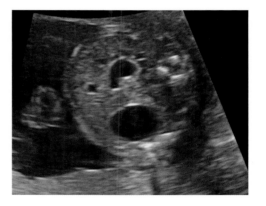

Obstetrics / Fetal Abnormalities

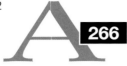

A. Duodenal atresia.

This image is a short-axis view of the fetal abdomen demonstrating two cystic structures with the appearance of a double bubble. The double bubble is a sign of duodenal atresia.

▶ Baun J: *Ob/Gyn Sonography: An Illustrated Review*. Pasadena, CA, Davies Publishing, 2016, p 232.

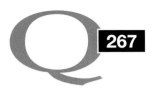

Absence of the fetal stomach on sonography could be suggestive of:

a. esophageal atresia
b. duodenal atresia
c. jejunal atresia
d. imperforate rectum

Obstetrics / Fetal Abnormalities

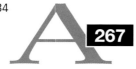

A. Esophageal atresia.

If the stomach is persistently absent, esophageal atresia may be present. The other choices listed would lead to dilated bowel, not an absent stomach. With esophageal atresia, polyhydramnios will be present.

▶ Baun J: *Ob/Gyn Sonography: An Illustrated Review*. Pasadena, CA, Davies Publishing, 2016, p 231.
▶ Gill KA: Anomalies associated with polyhydramnios. In Gill KA: *Ultrasound in Obstetrics and Gynecology: A Practitioner's Guide*. Pasadena, CA, Davies Publishing, 2014, pp 249–250.

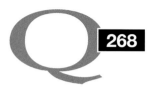

If the gallbladder is not visualized, the cause may be:

a. fetal hydrops
b. intrauterine growth restriction (IUGR)
c. erythroblastosis fetalis
d. cystic fibrosis

Obstetrics / Fetal Abnormalities

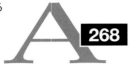

D. Cystic fibrosis.

Although the gallbladder is not routinely documented, absence of the fetal gallbladder may indicate cystic fibrosis (CF). If CF is suspected, the gallbladder should be documented.

▶ Rodriguez J, Gill KA: The second and third trimesters: basic and targeted scans. In Gill KA: *Ultrasound in Obstetrics and Gynecology: A Practitioner's Guide*. Pasadena, CA, Davies Publishing, 2014, p 136.

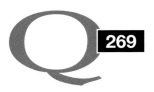

269

Which of the following conditions is most frequently associated with meconium ileus?

a. trisomy 13
b. trisomy 18
c. Potter sequence
d. cystic fibrosis

Obstetrics / Fetal Abnormalities

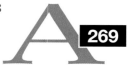

D. Cystic fibrosis.

Meconium ileus is the dilatation of the ileum after obstruction occurs. Fetuses with cystic fibrosis have a thickened meconium, and the ileum can rupture. Cystic fibrosis is typically a third trimester finding, although infrequently it can be seen in the second trimester.

- Abbott JF: The fetal abdominal wall and gastrointestinal tract. In Rumack CM (ed): *Diagnostic Ultrasound*, 4th edition. St. Louis, Mosby, 2011, pp 1327–1352.
- Baun J: *Ob/Gyn Sonography: An Illustrated Review*. Pasadena, CA, Davies Publishing, 2016, p 234.

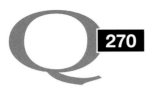

270

The narrowing of the hollow lumen of a segment of gut is called:

a. cloacal exstrophy
b. gastrointestinal ischemia
c. gastrointestinal atresia
d. caudal regression

Obstetrics / Fetal Abnormalities

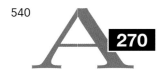

C. Gastrointestinal atresia.

Gastrointestinal atresia is a nonspecific term signifying narrowing of the intestinal tract.

▶ Baun J: *Ob/Gyn Sonography: An Illustrated Review*. Pasadena, CA, Davies Publishing, 2016, p 231.

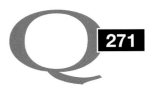

This image of the femur best demonstrates:

a. radial ray anomaly
b. homozygous achondroplasia
c. osteogenesis imperfecta
d. heterozygous achondroplasia

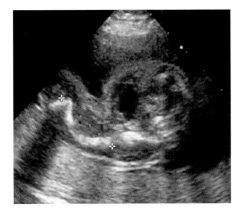

Obstetrics / Fetal Abnormalities

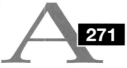

C. Osteogenesis imperfecta.

The curved femur seen in this image is suspicious for fracture, which can occur with type II osteogenesis imperfecta. Achondroplasias present with shortened long bones but without fractures. Radial ray anomaly is specific to the upper extremity.

▶ Baun J: *Ob/Gyn Sonography: An Illustrated Review*. Pasadena, CA, Davies Publishing, 2016, p 210.

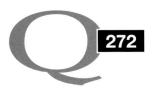

The nonlethal skeletal dysplasia characterized by mild rhizomelic shortening of the limbs and drop-off of femur length after 20 weeks is called:

a. achondroplasia
b. achondrogenesis
c. thanatophoric dysplasia
d. campomelic dysplasia

Obstetrics / Fetal Abnormalities

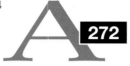

A. Achondroplasia.

Achondroplasia is an autosomal dominant nonlethal skeletal dysplasia characterized by rhizomelic limb shortening, frontal bossing, a flat nasal bridge, and a "trident-shaped" hand. *Achondrogenesis*, *thanatophoric dysplasia*, and *campomelic dysplasia* are typically lethal forms of dwarfism.

▶ Baun J: *Ob/Gyn Sonography: An Illustrated Review*. Pasadena, CA, Davies Publishing, 2016, pp 204–205.

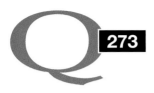

Q 273

Syndactyly is defined as the:

a. presence of extra digits on a single hand or foot
b. partial absence of a limb
c. absence of an extremity
d. soft tissue or bony fusion of digits

Obstetrics / Fetal Abnormalities

A **273**

D. Soft tissue or bony fusion of digits.

Syndactyly is fusion of the digits. Syndactyly may be as simple as webbed toes or as complicated as fusion of the bones of the adjacent fingers or toes.

▶ Baun J: *Ob/Gyn Sonography: An Illustrated Review*. Pasadena, CA, Davies Publishing, 2016, p 202.

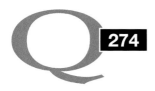

This image best demonstrates:

a. rocker bottom foot
b. talipes equinovarus
c. amniotic band sequence
d. radial ray anomaly

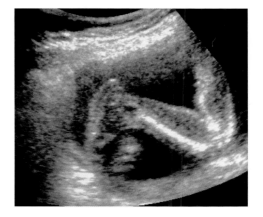

Obstetrics / Fetal Abnormalities

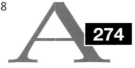

A. Rocker bottom foot.

This image is characteristic of rocker bottom foot, a finding that may be seen in trisomy 18.

▶ Baun J: *Ob/Gyn Sonography: An Illustrated Review*. Pasadena, CA, Davies Publishing, 2016, pp 213–214.

549

Abnormal congenital demineralization of fetal bony structure is called:

a. achondrogenesis
b. osteogenesis imperfecta
c. osteochondrodysplasia
d. campomelic dysplasia

Obstetrics / Fetal Abnormalities

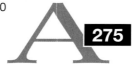

B. Osteogenesis imperfecta.

Osteogenesis imperfecta (OI) is a genetic condition characterized by extremely brittle bones caused by demineralization. In that respect OI is similar to hypophosphatasia. The type 2 form of OI is lethal and presents as multiple in utero long-bone fractures and decreased ossification of the skull.

▶ Baun J: *Ob/Gyn Sonography: An Illustrated Review*. Pasadena, CA, Davies Publishing, 2016, p 210.
▶ Callen PW: *Ultrasonography in Obstetrics and Gynecology*, 5th edition. Philadelphia, Elsevier, 2008, pp 156–158.

The presence of more than five digits on a single hand or foot is called:

a. syndactyly
b. mesomelia
c. rhizomelia
d. polydactyly

Obstetrics / Fetal Abnormalities

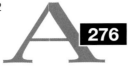

D. Polydactyly.

Polydactyly is the condition of extra digits on the hands or feet (*poly* means "many" or "more than usual"). *Syndactyly* means fused digits. *Rhizomelia* and *mesomelia*, respectively, describe shortening of the intermediate and proximal portions of the limbs.

▶ Baun J: *Ob/Gyn Sonography: An Illustrated Review*. Pasadena, CA, Davies Publishing, 2016, p 202.

Q 277

This image best demonstrates:

a. rocker bottom foot
b. amniotic band sequence
c. talipes equinovarus
d. radial ray anomaly

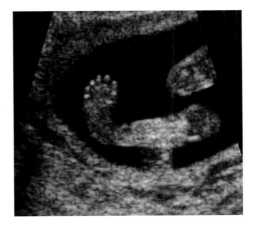

Obstetrics / Fetal Abnormalities

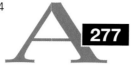

C. Talipes equinovarus.

This image is characteristic of clubfoot, also known as *talipes equinovarus*.

▶ Baun J: *Ob/Gyn Sonography: An Illustrated Review*. Pasadena, CA, Davies Publishing, 2016, pp 212–213.

A cloverleaf skull and a bell-shaped chest are two hallmark sonographic findings in which type of fetal skeletal abnormality?

a. short rib–polydactyly syndrome
b. campomelic dysplasia
c. chondrodysplasia punctata
d. thanatophoric dysplasia

Obstetrics / Fetal Abnormalities

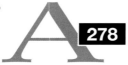

D. Thanatophoric dysplasia.

Thanatophoric dysplasia is a lethal skeletal dysplasia characterized by a cloverleaf-shaped skull and a narrowed thorax termed a *bell-shaped chest*. Death is usually due to respiratory failure because of the small chest.

▶ Baun J: *Ob/Gyn Sonography: An Illustrated Review*. Pasadena, CA, Davies Publishing, 2016, pp 205–206.

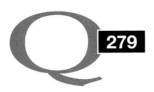

557

Congenital limb shortening that affects both proximal and distal segments of an extremity is called:

a. rhizomelia
b. micromelia
c. mesomelia
d. amelia

Obstetrics / Fetal Abnormalities

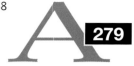

B. Micromelia.

With *micromelia* the limb is short in its entirety. *Rhizomelia* occurs when only the proximal part of the limb is short, and *mesomelia* when the mid portion is affected. With *amelia* the entire limb is absent.

▶ Baun J: *Ob/Gyn Sonography: An Illustrated Review*. Pasadena, CA, Davies Publishing, 2016, pp 203–204.

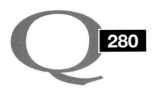

Hypoplasia of the middle phalanx of the fifth digit of the hand will cause:

a. syndactyly
b. clinodactyly
c. Down syndrome
d. adactyly

Obstetrics / Fetal Abnormalities

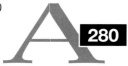

B. Clinodactyly.

The lack of or hypoplasia of the middle phalanx of the fifth digit causes the fifth digit to curve toward the fourth digit; such permanent lateral or medial deviation of a digit is called *clinodactyly*. Down syndrome is associated with (not caused by) hypoplasia of the middle phalanx of the fifth digit. *Syndactyly* is fusion of digits, and *adactyly* is absence of digits.

▶ Rodriguez J, Gill KA: The second and third trimesters: basic and targeted scans. In Gill KA: *Ultrasound in Obstetrics and Gynecology: A Practitioner's Guide*. Pasadena, CA, Davies Publishing, 2014, p 167.

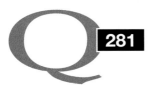

Q 281

Which of the following is considered to be a nonlethal fetal skeletal abnormality?

a. achondrogenesis
b. campomelic dysplasia
c. osteogenesis imperfecta type II
d. achondroplasia

Obstetrics / Fetal Abnormalities

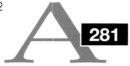

D. Achondroplasia.

Achondroplasia is the most common nonlethal type of skeletal dysplasia. With achondroplasia there is mild to moderate shortening of the femoral and humeral bone lengths. The other skeletal dysplasias listed are all lethal.

▸ Baun J: *Ob/Gyn Sonography: An Illustrated Review*. Pasadena, CA, Davies Publishing, 2016, pp 204–205.

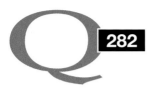

When a fetus is seen to have multiple joint contractures, one should suspect:

a. osteogenesis imperfecta
b. achondrogenesis
c. arthrogryposis
d. cubitus varus

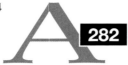

C. Arthrogryposis.

Arthrogryposis is a condition in which the fetal limbs are contracted and the fetus assumes a rigid posture. There are many causes of this condition, including oligohydramnios, genetic syndromes, and maternal conditions such as perinatal infection or hyperthermia. These images demonstrate the typical "praying mantis" position of the hands (top) and a fetal foot turned back on the leg (right).

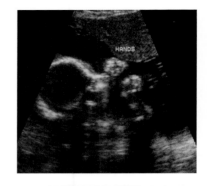

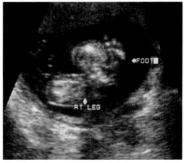

▶ Gill KA: Anomalies associated with polyhydramnios. In Gill KA: *Ultrasound in Obstetrics and Gynecology: A Practitioner's Guide*. Pasadena, CA, Davies Publishing, 2014, pp 256, 260.

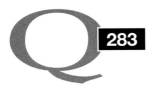

Q 283

Thanatophoric dwarfism has been associated with the:

a. strawberry-shaped head
b. cloverleaf-shaped head
c. lemon-shaped head
d. acrania

Obstetrics / Fetal Abnormalities

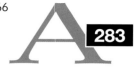

B. Cloverleaf-shaped head.

Thanatophoric dwarfism is associated with a cloverleaf-shaped skull, also referred to as *kleeblattschädel*. The strawberry shape is associated with trisomy 18 and the lemon shape is associated with the Arnold-Chiari malformation (Chiari malformation type II). Acrania is a brain without a skull.

- Baun J: *Ob/Gyn Sonography: An Illustrated Review*. Pasadena, CA, Davies Publishing, 2016, pp 205–206.
- Gill KA: Anomalies associated with polyhydramnios. In Gill KA: *Ultrasound in Obstetrics and Gynecology: A Practitioner's Guide*. Pasadena, CA, Davies Publishing, 2014, p 258.

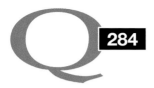

This long-axis image of a second trimester fetus obtained from a 40-year-old patient suggests the following diagnosis:

a. intrauterine growth restriction (IUGR)
b. osteogenesis imperfecta
c. thanatophoric dysplasia
d. achondroplasia

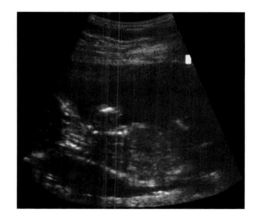

Obstetrics / Fetal Abnormalities

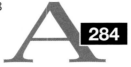

C. Thanatophoric dysplasia.

Thanatophoric dysplasia is a lethal form of skeletal dysplasia characterized by bowed long bones, a narrow thorax, and a large cloverleaf-shaped skull. Most cases present with polyhydramnios. The very narrow thorax is the key finding in this image.

▶ Baun J: *Ob/Gyn Sonography: An Illustrated Review*. Pasadena, CA, Davies Publishing, 2016, pp 205–206.
▶ Gill KA: Anomalies associated with polyhydramnios. In Gill KA: *Ultrasound in Obstetrics and Gynecology: A Practitioner's Guide*. Pasadena, CA, Davies Publishing, 2014, pp 258–259.

285

Rhizomelia indicates abnormal shortening of which of the following long bones?

a. radius
b. humerus
c. ulna
d. tibia

285

B. Humerus.

Rhizomelia is abnormal shortening of the proximal long bones, such as the humerus or femur. With *micromelia* the entire limb is shortened. *Mesomelia* is shortening of only the distal portion of the limb, such as the radius, ulna, or tibia.

▶ Baun J: *Ob/Gyn Sonography: An Illustrated Review*. Pasadena, CA, Davies Publishing, 2016, p 201.

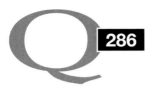

571

What is the name of the congenital cardiac anomaly characterized by the aorta arising from the right ventricle and the pulmonary trunk arising from the left ventricle?

a. transposition of the great vessels
b. tetralogy of Fallot
c. conotruncal abnormality
d. persistent truncus arteriosus

Obstetrics / Fetal Abnormalities

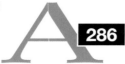

A. Transposition of the great vessels.

With *transposition of the great vessels* (TGV, also known as *transposition of the great arteries*, TGA), the normal anatomic positions of the aorta and pulmonary artery are reversed, with the aorta arising from the right ventricle and the pulmonary artery arising from the left ventricle. In a corrected transposition, the ventricles are switched too. This condition constitutes 3% of congenital heart defects and is the most common cause of "blue baby syndrome."

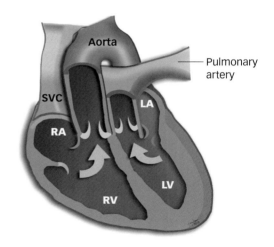

▶ Baun J: *Ob/Gyn Sonography: An Illustrated Review*. Pasadena, CA, Davies Publishing, 2016, pp 177–178.

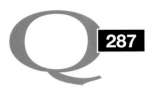

287

What is the name of the rare congenital chest anomaly in which all or part of the heart is located outside of the thoracic cavity?

a. Ebstein's anomaly
b. diaphragmatic hernia
c. ectopia cordis
d. omphalocele

Obstetrics / Fetal Abnormalities

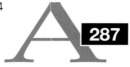

C. Ectopia cordis.

In *ectopia cordis* the fetal heart is located external to the thorax. When this anomaly appears with omphalocele and other associated anomalies, it is termed *pentalogy of Cantrell.*

▶ Baun J: *Ob/Gyn Sonography: An Illustrated Review*. Pasadena, CA, Davies Publishing, 2016, p 186.

What is the most common congenital cardiac anomaly?

a. tetralogy of Fallot
b. ventricular septal defect
c. atrial septal defect
d. aortic coarctation

Obstetrics / Fetal Abnormalities

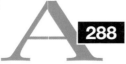

B. Ventricular septal defect.

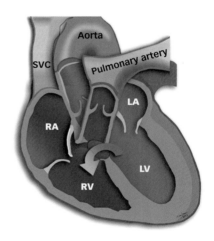

A *ventricular septal defect* (VSD) is an abnormal communication between the right (RV) and left (LV) ventricles through a defect in the interventricular septum (curved arrow). It is the most common congenital cardiac anomaly, occurring in about 1 in 400 live births, and can appear either as an isolated abnormality or in association with other cardiac anomalies. RA = right atrium, LA = left atrium, SVC = superior vena cava.

▶ Baun J: *Ob/Gyn Sonography: An Illustrated Review*. Pasadena, CA, Davies Publishing, 2016, p 173.

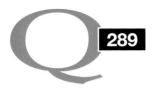

What anomaly is demonstrated in this image?

a. transposition of great vessels
b. patent ductus arteriosus
c. aortic coarctation
d. pulmonary stenosis

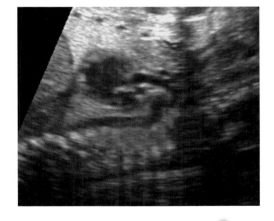

Obstetrics / Fetal Abnormalities

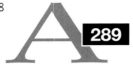

C. Aortic coarctation.

This image presents an anomalous aortic arch, consistent with aortic coarctation. The aorta appears to be arising from the center of the heart, ruling out transposition. The ductus arteriosus and pulmonary artery are not visible in this image for evaluation.

▶ Baun J: *Ob/Gyn Sonography: An Illustrated Review*. Pasadena, CA, Davies Publishing, 2016, p 184.

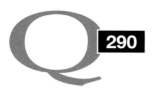

Q 290

Ebstein's anomaly is characterized primarily by:

a. tricuspid valve displaced inferiorly in the right ventricle
b. mitral valve displaced inferiorly in the left ventricle
c. overriding aorta
d. all or part of the heart located outside the thoracic cavity

Obstetrics / Fetal Abnormalities

A 290

A. Tricuspid valve displaced inferiorly in the right ventricle.

Ebstein's anomaly is a tricuspid valve that is too inferiorly located in the right ventricle. In other words, it is too close to the apex. This causes an enlarged right ventricle and marked tricuspid regurgitation.

▶ Baun J: *Ob/Gyn Sonography: An Illustrated Review*. Pasadena, CA, Davies Publishing, 2016, pp 182–183.

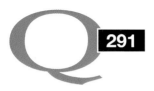
291

Of the following fetal cardiac anomalies, which can be easily missed on the four-chamber view?

a. situs inversus
b. transposition of the great vessels
c. Ebstein's anomaly
d. hypoplastic left ventricle

Obstetrics / Fetal Abnormalities

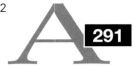

B. Transposition of the great vessels.

It is possible to have a normal four-chamber view of the fetal heart in the presence of transposition of the great vessels (TGV). The crossing of the outflow tracts rules out TGV. Determination of left versus right ventricle is made easier by visualization of the moderator band, which exists only in the morphologic right ventricle. In the presence of any of the other choices, the four-chamber view of the fetal heart would be abnormal.

▶ Baun J: *Ob/Gyn Sonography: An Illustrated Review*. Pasadena, CA, Davies Publishing, 2016, pp 162–165.
▶ Rodriguez J, Gill KA: The second and third trimesters: basic and targeted scans. In Gill KA: *Ultrasound in Obstetrics and Gynecology: A Practitioner's Guide*. Pasadena, CA, Davies Publishing, 2014, p 155.

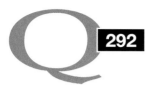

This M-mode image demonstrates that the heart rate of this second trimester fetus is:

a. normal
b. irregular
c. tachycardic
d. bradycardic

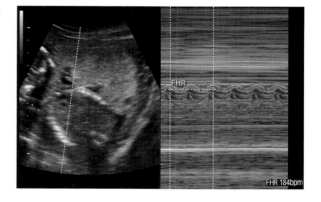

Obstetrics / Fetal Abnormalities

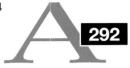

C. Tachycardic.

A normal second trimester fetal heart rate is between 100 and 180 bpm. The M-mode image identifies the fetal heart rate as 184 bpm, which is in the tachycardic range.

- Baun J: *Ob/Gyn Sonography: An Illustrated Review*. Pasadena, CA, Davies Publishing, 2016, p 189.
- Rodriguez J, Gill KA: The second and third trimesters: basic and targeted scans. In Gill KA: *Ultrasound in Obstetrics and Gynecology: A Practitioner's Guide*. Pasadena, CA, Davies Publishing, 2014, p 128.

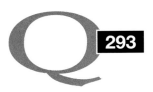

293

In which of these vessels will flow be reversed in the presence of tricuspid regurgitation?

a. umbilical artery
b. ductus venosus
c. middle cerebral artery
d. ductus arteriosus

Obstetrics / Fetal Abnormalities

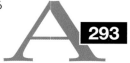

A 293

B. Ductus venosus.

The *ductus venosus* (DV) is a regulator of oxygen to the fetus, opening and closing as necessary to shunt blood directly to the fetal heart in the event of fetal compromise. The DV is connected to the inferior vena cava (IVC), which is connected to the right atrium. Normally, the ductus venosus has forward flow toward the heart. Tricuspid regurgitation causes back pressure, resulting in reversal of flow in the ductus venosus.

▶ Gill KA: *Ultrasound in Obstetrics and Gynecology: A Practitioner's Guide*. Pasadena, CA, Davies Publishing, p 388.

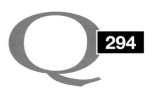

Which spectral Doppler control adjusts the number of heartbeats displayed on the screen at one time?

a. spectral gain
b. baseline
c. scale
d. sweep speed

Obstetrics / Fetal Abnormalities

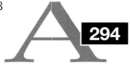

D. Sweep speed.

The sweep speed control can be adjusted so that fewer heartbeats are displayed on the screen, which is useful for measuring parameters such as acceleration. Sweep speed may also be adjusted so more heartbeats are displayed, which is useful when identifying arrhythmias.

▶ Raatz Stephenson S (ed): *Diagnostic Medical Sonography: Obstetrics and Gynecology*, 3rd edition. Baltimore, Lippincott Williams & Wilkins, 2012, ch 19.

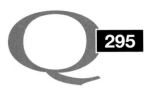

295

Uncontrolled diabetes mellitus can lead to sirenomelia, a severe fetal anomaly also associated with:

a. rachischisis
b. caudal regression syndrome
c. spina bifida occulta
d. anencephaly

Obstetrics / Fetal Abnormalities

A **295**

B. Caudal regression syndrome.

Sirenomelia (also known as *mermaid syndrome*) is a severe form of caudal regression syndrome, which occurs more commonly when the mother is an insulin-dependent diabetic (IDDM). *Caudal regression syndrome* is caused by a defect during embryogenesis that leads to failure of the caudal portion of the fetus to develop. The other conditions listed are not specific to cases of IDDM mothers. Although the other choices listed are neural tube defects, only sirenomelia is specific to caudal regression syndrome.

▶ Baun J: *Ob/Gyn Sonography: An Illustrated Review*. Pasadena, CA, Davies Publishing, 2016, p 290.

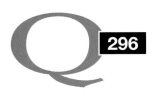

A normal range for nuchal translucency measured between weeks 11 and 14 is:

a. 1.0–2.5 mm
b. 1.0–4.0 mm
c. 1.5–3.5 mm
d. 1.0–3.0 mm

Obstetrics / Fetal Abnormalities

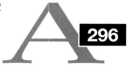

A. 1.0–2.5 mm.

Nuchal translucency refers to the collection of lymphatic fluid found in the posterior neck region of the embryo, which is normal in early pregnancy but can indicate genetic anomalies if it exceeds normal values. From menstrual weeks 11 to 14, the normal nuchal translucency is 1.0 to 2.5 mm. Because the range is so small, care must be taken to avoid error, which is common. High-resolution magnification is used to ensure correct caliper placement that includes only the area of sonolucent thickening posterior to the fetal neck and excludes the soft tissue adjacent to this space. The nuchal translucency is typically not measured when the crown-rump length (CRL) exceeds 84 mm. (See also the answer to question 140.)

- Baun J: *Ob/Gyn Sonography: An Illustrated Review*. Pasadena, CA, Davies Publishing, 2016, pp 13, 276–277.
- Rodriguez J, Gill KA: The second and third trimesters: basic and targeted scans. In Gill KA: *Ultrasound in Obstetrics and Gynecology: A Practitioner's Guide*. Pasadena, CA, Davies Publishing, 2014, pp 142–143.

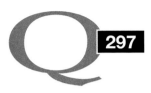

The normal nuchal fold thickness should not exceed:

a. 2–3 mm
b. 3–4 mm
c. 4–5 mm
d. 5–6 mm

Obstetrics / Fetal Abnormalities

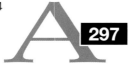

D. 5–6 mm.

> The best answer is D. Some sources state that any nuchal fold thickness greater than 6 mm is abnormal, while others now consider nuchal fold thickness greater than 5 mm to be abnormal and still others consider the threshold to be greater than 5–6 mm. Any measurement 5 mm or greater should be brought to the attention of the interpreting physician. It is important to note the distinction between *nuchal translucency* (measured between 11 and 14 weeks) and *nuchal fold thickness*, which is usually measured between 15 and 20 menstrual weeks and typically not after 20–21 weeks. (See also the answer to question 139.)

▶ Baun J: *Ob/Gyn Sonography: An Illustrated Review*. Pasadena, CA, Davies Publishing, 2016, p 278.
▶ Rodriguez J, Gill KA: The second and third trimesters: basic and targeted scans. In Gill KA: *Ultrasound in Obstetrics and Gynecology: A Practitioner's Guide*. Pasadena, CA, Davies Publishing, 2014, p 144.

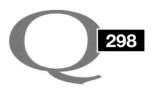

298

Measurement of the nuchal fold thickness is taken at the level of the:

a. thalami
b. falx
c. third ventricle
d. cerebellum

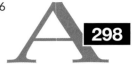

D. Cerebellum.

The nuchal skin fold is measured from an axial oblique section through the fetal head at the level of the posterior fossa, including the cerebellum and the cisterna magna. Calipers should be placed on the outer edge of the occipital bone and the outer edge of the overlying soft tissue.

- Baun J: *Ob/Gyn Sonography: An Illustrated Review*. Pasadena, CA, Davies Publishing, 2016, p 278.
- Rodriguez J, Gill KA: The second and third trimesters: basic and targeted scans. In Gill KA: *Ultrasound in Obstetrics and Gynecology: A Practitioner's Guide*. Pasadena, CA, Davies Publishing, 2014, p 144.

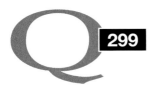

This fetus had choroid plexus cysts along with the finding seen in this image. What is the most likely diagnosis given these findings?

a. trisomy 18
b. triploidy
c. trisomy 13
d. trisomy 21

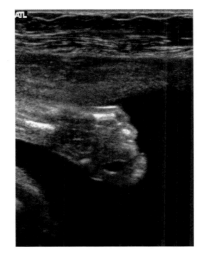

Obstetrics / Fetal Abnormalities / AIT—PACSim

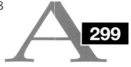

A. Trisomy 18.

This is an image of *clinodactyly*, which is an overlapping finger or inward curvature of a digit, a finding that may be found in fetuses with trisomy 18. Although clinodactyly is not specific to trisomy 18, the association with choroid plexus cysts makes it more likely that the fetus is affected with trisomy 18.

- Baun J: *Ob/Gyn Sonography: An Illustrated Review*. Pasadena, CA, Davies Publishing, 2016, pp 284–285.
- Gill KA: Fetal syndromes. In Gill KA: *Ultrasound in Obstetrics and Gynecology: A Practitioner's Guide*. Pasadena, CA, Davies Publishing, 2014, p 349.

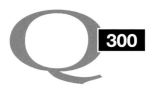

The sonographic abnormality demonstrated in this image is more commonly associated with which of the following syndromes?

a. tetralogy of Fallot
b. VACTERL association
c. CHARGE association
d. pentalogy of Cantrell

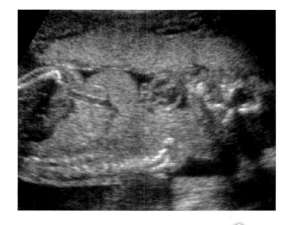

Obstetrics / Fetal Abnormalities

A 300

D. Pentalogy of Cantrell.

Pentalogy of Cantrell is five separate anomalies, one of which is ectopia cordis, seen in the image. *Tetralogy of Fallot* is a combination of heart defects. *VACTERL* stands for vertebral, anal, cardiac, tracheoesophageal, renal, and limb—the body parts affected in a fetus with this association. *CHARGE* stands for coloboma of the eye, heart defects, atresia of the nasal choanae, retardation of growth and/or development, genital and/or urinary abnormalities, and ear abnormalities and deafness.

▶ Baun J: *Ob/Gyn Sonography: An Illustrated Review*. Pasadena, CA, Davies Publishing, 2016, pp 292–293.

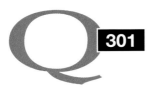

Q 301

Trisomy 18 is also called:

a. Edwards syndrome
b. Down syndrome
c. Patau syndrome
d. Meckel-Gruber syndrome

Obstetrics / Fetal Abnormalities

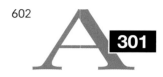

A. Edwards syndrome.

The other name for trisomy 18 is *Edwards syndrome*.

▶ Baun J: *Ob/Gyn Sonography: An Illustrated Review*. Pasadena, CA, Davies Publishing, 2016, pp 284–285.

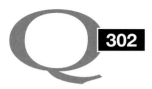

Q 302

Trisomy 21 is also known as:

a. Patau syndrome
b. Edwards syndrome
c. Down syndrome
d. Turner syndrome

Obstetrics / Fetal Abnormalities

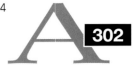

C. Down syndrome.

Trisomy 21 is also known as *Down syndrome*. Trisomy 18 is also known as *Edwards syndrome*, and trisomy 13 is also known as *Patau syndrome*. *Trisomy* implies an extra chromosome (three as opposed to the normal two).

- Baun J: *Ob/Gyn Sonography: An Illustrated Review*. Pasadena, CA, Davies Publishing, 2016, pp 283–284.
- Gill KA: Fetal syndromes. In Gill KA: *Ultrasound in Obstetrics and Gynecology: A Practitioner's Guide*. Pasadena, CA, Davies Publishing, 2014, pp 351–352.

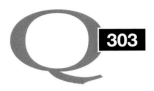

Q 303

The triad of infantile polycystic kidneys, a posterior encephalocele, and polydactyly suggests:

a. Eagle-Barrett syndrome
b. Potter sequence
c. Arnold-Chiari syndrome
d. Meckel-Gruber syndrome

Obstetrics / Fetal Abnormalities

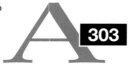

D. Meckel-Gruber syndrome.

Meckel-Gruber syndrome (also known as *dysencephalia splanchnocystica* or simply *Meckel syndrome*) is characterized by bilateral enlarged polycystic kidneys (always), posterior encephalocele (80%), and polydactyly (75%). Eagle-Barrett is prune belly syndrome, Potter sequence is severe oligohydramnios from renal disease or agenesis, and Arnold-Chiari is a series of findings in a fetus with a myelomeningocele.

▶ Baun J: *Ob/Gyn Sonography: An Illustrated Review*. Pasadena, CA, Davies Publishing, 2016, pp 291–292.
▶ Gill KA: Fetal syndromes. In Gill KA: *Ultrasound in Obstetrics and Gynecology: A Practitioner's Guide*. Pasadena, CA, Davies Publishing, 2014, pp 358–359.

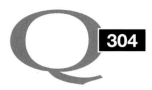

607

304

What is another name for the congenital genetic condition in which one of the sex chromosomes is absent while the other is an X chromosome (otherwise known as *XO syndrome*)?

a. Down syndrome
b. Edwards syndrome
c. Turner syndrome
d. Meckel-Gruber syndrome

Obstetrics / Fetal Abnormalities

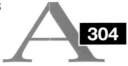

C. Turner syndrome.

With Turner syndrome (also known as 45,X) there is only a single sex chromosome, which is female (X), instead of two sex chromosomes. Turner syndrome is identified in utero most often by the presence of a cystic hygroma. A child affected with Turner syndrome is phenotypically female with a webbed neck and "streak" (nonfunctional) ovaries.

▶ Baun J: *Ob/Gyn Sonography: An Illustrated Review*. Pasadena, CA, Davies Publishing, 2016, 286–287.

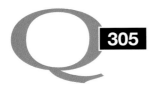

The area on the posterior surface of this 11-week fetus demonstrates:

a. increased nuchal translucency
b. nuchal fold thickening
c. cystic hygroma
d. a normal amnion close to the fetus

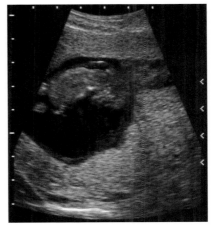

Obstetrics / Fetal Abnormalities

A 305

A. Increased nuchal translucency.

Increased nuchal translucency is associated with chromosomal anomalies such as trisomy 21, as well as cardiac defects. Nuchal translucency is measured between 11 and 14 weeks; nuchal fold thickness, between 15 and 20 weeks. (See also the answers to questions 139, 140, 296, 297, and 298.)

▶ Baun J: *Ob/Gyn Sonography: An Illustrated Review*. Pasadena, CA, Davies Publishing, 2016, p 277.
▶ Gill KA: Fetal syndromes. In Gill KA: *Ultrasound in Obstetrics and Gynecology: A Practitioner's Guide*. Pasadena, CA, Davies Publishing, 2014, p 354.

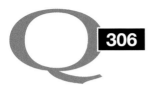

What does this image demonstrate?

a. It shows an image of normal anatomy.
b. It shows abnormal brain development.
c. It shows a cranial abnormality.
d. It shows a fetus at risk for aneuploidy.

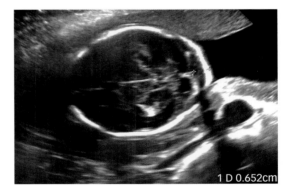

Obstetrics / Fetal Abnormalities

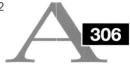

D. It shows a fetus at risk for aneuploidy.

This image demonstrates a thickened nuchal fold, greater than 6 mm (or, according to some authorities, greater than 5 mm), which is a marker for aneuploidy, such as trisomy 21. The rest of the image is unremarkable. See also the answer to question 297.

▶ Baun J: *Ob/Gyn Sonography: An Illustrated Review*. Pasadena, CA, Davies Publishing, 2016, p 278.
▶ Gill KA: Fetal syndromes. In Gill KA: *Ultrasound in Obstetrics and Gynecology: A Practitioner's Guide*. Pasadena, CA, Davies Publishing, 2014, pp 353–354.

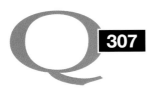

307

This image of the right forearm and hand of a 20-week fetus is suspicious for:

a. clubhand
b. polydactyly
c. ectrodactyly
d. radial ray anomaly

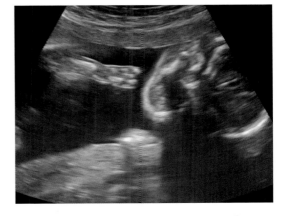

Obstetrics / Fetal Abnormalities

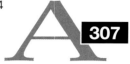

D. Radial ray anomaly.

This image shows an abnormal forearm and missing digits, consistent with a form of *radial ray anomaly*. *Clubhand* (*talipomanus*) presents as a hand that is abnormally rotated inward. *Ectrodactyly* is a "lobster claw" or split-hand anomaly with fused or absent digits. *Polydactyly* is the condition of having extra digits.

▶ Baun J: *Ob/Gyn Sonography: An Illustrated Review*. Pasadena, CA, Davies Publishing, 2016, p 212.

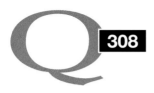

Which of the following conditions may involve defects of the heart, limbs, vertebrae, and kidneys as well as anal atresia and tracheoesophageal fistula?

a. Ellis–van Creveld syndrome
b. VACTERL association
c. Holt-Oram syndrome
d. Meckel-Gruber syndrome

Obstetrics / Fetal Abnormalities

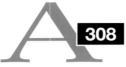

B. VACTERL association.

VACTERL stands for vertebral defects, anal atresia, cardiac defects, tracheoesophageal fistula, renal anomalies, and limb abnormalities. It is a collection of clinical features that point to other, less apparent abnormalities—known as an *association* (as opposed to a syndrome).

- Baun J: *Ob/Gyn Sonography: An Illustrated Review*. Pasadena, CA, Davies Publishing, 2016, p 293.
- Gill KA: Anomalies associated with polyhydramnios. In Gill KA: *Ultrasound in Obstetrics and Gynecology: A Practitioner's Guide*. Pasadena, CA, Davies Publishing, 2014, p 255.

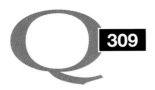

The sonographic abnormality demonstrated in this image is more commonly associated with which of the following fetal conditions?

a. amniotic band sequence
b. VACTERL association
c. caudal regression syndrome
d. CHARGE association

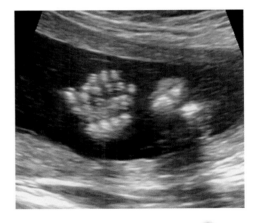

Obstetrics / Fetal Abnormalities

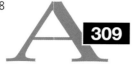

B. VACTERL association.

The limb anomaly, in this case polydactyly, indicates that it may be part of an association of anomalies. There are several such associations. *VACTERL* includes vertebral defects, anal atresia, cardiac defects, tracheoesophageal fistula, renal anomalies, and limb abnormalities. *CHARGE* is another association, including coloboma of the eye, heart defects, atresia of the nasal choanae, growth restriction, genital and/or urinary abnormalities, and ear abnormalities and deafness. *Caudal regression* and *amniotic band* cause deletion of body parts, not extra body parts.

▶ Baun J: *Ob/Gyn Sonography: An Illustrated Review*. Pasadena, CA, Davies Publishing, 2016, pp 293–294.

Which of the following associations includes genitourinary anomalies, heart defects, ear and eye problems, and growth restriction?

a. amniotic band sequence
b. VACTERL association
c. caudal regression syndrome
d. CHARGE association

Obstetrics / Fetal Abnormalities

A 310

D. CHARGE association.

CHARGE is an association including coloboma of the eye, heart defects, atresia of the nasal choanae, restriction of growth and/or development, genital and/or urinary abnormalities, and ear abnormalities and deafness.

▶ Baun J: *Ob/Gyn Sonography: An Illustrated Review*. Pasadena, CA, Davies Publishing, 2016, pp 293–294.

How does estrogen affect coexisting fibroids during pregnancy?

a. It causes fibroid growth.
b. It slows the growth of fibroids.
c. It causes degeneration of fibroids.
d. It causes additional fibroids to form.

Obstetrics / Coexisting Disorders

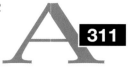

A. It causes fibroid growth.

Estrogen may cause fibroid growth, so fibroids are typically examined during pregnancy for size. Fibroids that outgrow their blood supply may degenerate, which may be a source of pain for the patient.

- Baun J: *Ob/Gyn Sonography: An Illustrated Review*. Pasadena, CA, Davies Publishing, 2016, pp 328–329, 376.
- Gill KA: Maternal disorders and pregnancy. In Gill KA: *Ultrasound in Obstetrics and Gynecology: A Practitioner's Guide*. Pasadena, CA, Davies Publishing, 2014, p 330.

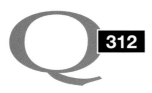

312

What type of cyst is formed when a follicle does not rupture and release the ovum?

a. theca-lutein cyst
b. cystadenoma
c. cystic teratoma
d. follicular cyst

Obstetrics / Coexisting Disorders

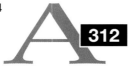

D. Follicular cyst.

Follicular cysts result from failure of ovulation. The growing cyst may be a source of pain as it can grow to more than 5 cm. *Cystadenomas* and *cystic teratomas* are other ovarian masses, and *theca-lutein cysts* are associated with gestational trophoblastic disease.

- Baun J: *Ob/Gyn Sonography: An Illustrated Review*. Pasadena, CA, Davies Publishing, 2016, pp 384–385.
- Gill KA: Introduction to diagnostic ultrasound. In Gill KA: *Ultrasound in Obstetrics and Gynecology: A Practitioner's Guide*. Pasadena, CA, Davies Publishing, 2014, pp 56–57.

Which of the following ovarian pathologies is associated with hydatidiform mole?

a. theca-lutein cysts
b. corpus luteum cysts
c. follicular cysts
d. paraovarian cysts

Obstetrics / Coexisting Disorders

A 313

A. Theca-lutein cysts.

Theca-lutein cysts are large cysts on the ovaries that coexist with hydatidiform mole. The other cysts may occur but are not specific to molar pregnancies.

▶ Baun J: *Ob/Gyn Sonography: An Illustrated Review*. Pasadena, CA, Davies Publishing, 2016, pp 20–21.

The sonographic findings in this image are most consistent with:

a. complete hydatidiform mole
b. partial hydatidiform mole
c. chorioadenoma destruens
d. placental abruption

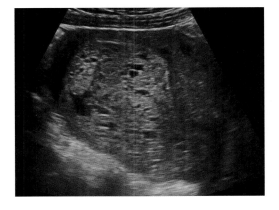

Obstetrics / Coexisting Disorders

A 314

A. Complete hydatidiform mole.

Complete hydatidiform mole presents with a "bunch of grapes" appearance. Clinically, the patient may have hyperemesis gravidarum, bleeding, and a markedly high beta-hCG level.

▶ Baun J: *Ob/Gyn Sonography: An Illustrated Review*. Pasadena, CA, Davies Publishing, 2016, p 20.

What is the name of the pathologic entity in which an intrauterine gestation is composed completely of multisized hydropic villi?

a. cornual pregnancy
b. anembryonic pregnancy
c. hydatidiform mole
d. hydropic degeneration of placenta

Obstetrics / Coexisting Disorders

A 315

C. Hydatidiform mole.

Hydatidiform mole is a pregnancy failure that most commonly occurs when a sperm cell fertilizes an anucleate egg. An abnormal growth of villous trophoblastic tissue causes vesicles to fill the uterine canal, resulting in the classic "bunch of grapes" appearance on ultrasound.

▶ Baun J: *Ob/Gyn Sonography: An Illustrated Review*. Pasadena, CA, Davies Publishing, 2016, p 20.
▶ Callen PW: *Ultrasonography in Obstetrics and Gynecology*, 5th edition. Philadelphia, Elsevier, 2008, p 951.

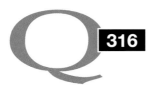

This patient presents large for gestational age and bleeding. Her pregnancy titers are extremely high. No fetal heart tones can be heard. Judging from this transverse image through the uterus, the diagnosis is most likely:

a. ectopic pregnancy
b. incomplete abortion
c. twin demise
d. molar pregnancy

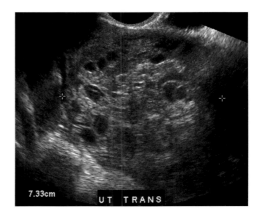

Obstetrics / Coexisting Disorders / AIT—PACSim

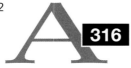

D. Molar pregnancy.

The patient's symptoms and evidence in this image present a classic history for a molar pregnancy.

- Baun J: *Ob/Gyn Sonography: An Illustrated Review*. Pasadena, CA, Davies Publishing, 2016, pp 20–22.
- Sliman MH, Gill KA: The first trimester. In Gill KA: *Ultrasound in Obstetrics and Gynecology: A Practitioner's Guide*. Pasadena, CA, Davies Publishing, 2014, pp 111–113.

A patient presents with a history of a hydatidiform mole evacuated 3 months prior. Routine serum surveillance demonstrates a sudden increase in beta-hCG levels. This image raises suspicions for:

a. Stein-Leventhal syndrome
b. recurrent trophoblastic disease
c. retained molar tissue
d. abdominal abscess

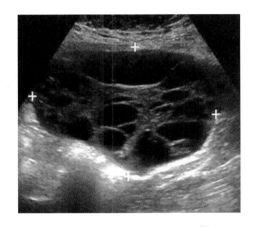

Obstetrics / Coexisting Disorders / AIT—PACSim

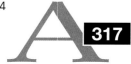

B. Recurrent trophoblastic disease.

After evacuation of a molar pregnancy, beta-hCG levels should be checked for recurrent mole. Given the patient history, the lab values, and what appears to be a theca-lutein cyst on ultrasound, recurrent mole should be suspected.

▶ Baun J: *Ob/Gyn Sonography: An Illustrated Review*. Pasadena, CA, Davies Publishing, 2016, pp 22–23.

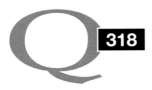

This image best demonstrates:

a. spina bifida
b. limb–body wall complex
c. external sacrococcygeal teratoma
d. presacral teratoma

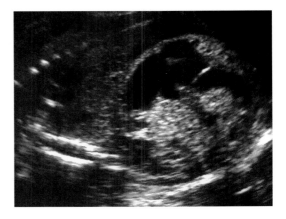

Obstetrics / Coexisting Disorders

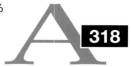

D. Presacral teratoma.

There are four types of sacrococcygeal teratomas, ranging from completely external (type I) to completely internal (presacral, type IV). This image shows a large, complex fetal abdominopelvic mass that appears to be completely internal.

▶ Baun J: *Ob/Gyn Sonography: An Illustrated Review*. Pasadena, CA, Davies Publishing, 2016, pp 240–241.
▶ Gill KA: Anomalies associated with polyhydramnios. In Gill KA: *Ultrasound in Obstetrics and Gynecology: A Practitioner's Guide*. Pasadena, CA, Davies Publishing, 2014, pp 241–242.

The most common site for a fetal teratoma is the:

a. face
b. sacrococcygeal region
c. neck
d. mediastinum

Obstetrics / Coexisting Disorders

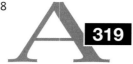

B. Sacrococcygeal region.

Sacrococcygeal teratomas are the most common tumor seen in newborns. Teratomas may occur in the fetal face as well as other locations.

▶ Baun J: *Ob/Gyn Sonography: An Illustrated Review*. Pasadena, CA, Davies Publishing, 2016, p 103.
▶ Gill KA: Anomalies associated with polyhydramnios. In Gill KA: *Ultrasound in Obstetrics and Gynecology: A Practitioner's Guide*. Pasadena, CA, Davies Publishing, 2014, p 240.

This mass was seen extending off the inferior aspect of the fetal spine. A spinal defect could not be observed and no other anomalies were seen. The most likely diagnosis would be:

a. lumbar myelomeningocele
b. sacrococcygeal teratoma
c. anal prolapse
d. bladder exstrophy

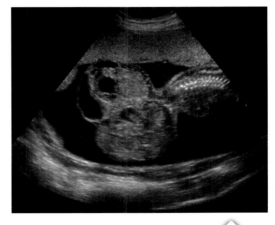

Obstetrics / Coexisting Disorders / AIT—PACSim

A **320**

B. Sacrococcygeal teratoma.

This image presents a fetus with a large complex mass external to the fetal rump. Given the history of a normal-appearing spine, this mass is most likely a sacrococcygeal teratoma.

▶ Baun J: *Ob/Gyn Sonography: An Illustrated Review*. Pasadena, CA, Davies Publishing, 2016, pp 142, 241–242.
▶ Gill KA: Anomalies associated with polyhydramnios. In Gill KA: *Ultrasound in Obstetrics and Gynecology: A Practitioner's Guide*. Pasadena, CA, Davies Publishing, 2014, pp 241–242.

321

Which of the following is the best way to differentiate a leiomyoma from focal uterine contraction?

a. Examine using spectral Doppler.
b. Have the patient fill the urinary bladder.
c. Perform amniocentesis.
d. Reevaluate after 30 minutes.

Obstetrics / Coexisting Disorders

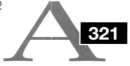

D. Reevaluate after 30 minutes.

Unlike focal uterine contractions, leiomyomas do not go away with time. Although color Doppler may be helpful, spectral Doppler will not help in this case.

- Baun J: *Ob/Gyn Sonography: An Illustrated Review*. Pasadena, CA, Davies Publishing, 2016, pp 328–329.
- Callen PW: *Ultrasonography in Obstetrics and Gynecology*, 5th edition. Philadelphia, Elsevier, 2008, p 1104.

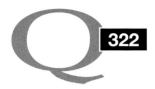

643

In this image, myometrial contractions in the lower uterine segment (LUS) are mimicking:

a. placental abruption
b. placental mass
c. funneled cervix
d. vasa previa

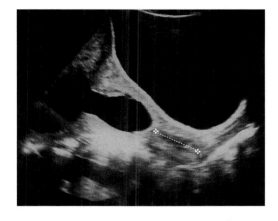

Obstetrics / Coexisting Disorders

A **322**

C. Funneled cervix.

This image presents a normal-length cervix with LUS myometrial contractions mimicking funneling of the cervix. Myometrial contractions can also mimic a placental mass, but not in the image provided.

▶ Gill KA: *Ultrasound in Obstetrics and Gynecology: A Practitioner's Guide*. Pasadena, CA, Davies Publishing, 2014, p 217.

Which of the following is a serious complication of ovarian masses in pregnancy?

a. torsion
b. spontaneous abortion
c. placental abruption
d. premature labor

Obstetrics / Coexisting Disorders

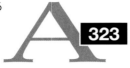

A. Torsion.

Ovarian masses can torse the ovary as the uterus grows with pregnancy and displaces the ovaries. Ovarian torsion is a surgical emergency.

- Baun J: *Ob/Gyn Sonography: An Illustrated Review*. Pasadena, CA, Davies Publishing, 2016, p 397.
- Gill KA: Introduction to diagnostic ultrasound. In Gill KA: *Ultrasound in Obstetrics and Gynecology: A Practitioner's Guide*. Pasadena, CA, Davies Publishing, 2014, pp 64–65.

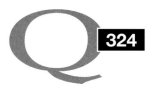

324

Your patient will need to deliver by cesarean section if she has undergone which of the following procedures?

a. McDonald's procedure
b. Valsalva maneuver
c. digital examination
d. transabdominal cerclage

Obstetrics / Coexisting Disorders

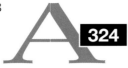

D. Transabdominal cerclage.

A *transabdominal cerclage* is placed at the uterine isthmus, higher than a vaginal cerclage. A transabdominal cerclage is permanent and is not removed, necessitating a c-section. Although a *McDonald's procedure* is a type of vaginal cerclage, it does not require a c-section delivery because the stitch is placed on the lower cervix and can easily be removed. A *Valsalva maneuver* is a bearing down on abdominal muscles as if one were trying to have a bowel movement. A *digital examination* is performed by a clinician to palpate the cervix.

- Cunningham FG, Leveno KJ, Bloom SL, et al: *Williams Obstetrics*, 24th edition. New York, McGraw-Hill, 2014, p 363.
- Foy PM: Ultrasound of the cervix during pregnancy. In Gill KA: *Ultrasound in Obstetrics and Gynecology: A Practitioner's Guide*. Pasadena, CA, Davies Publishing, 2014, pp 218–219.

325

A live fetus is seen in a gestational sac with a large, hydropic, cystic-appearing placenta. Which of the following is most likely?

a. triploidy
b. normal pregnancy
c. Down syndrome
d. intrauterine growth restriction

Obstetrics / Coexisting Disorders

A 325

A. Triploidy.

A live fetus with a large, hydropic placenta is consistent with partial mole. With partial mole the fetus is usually triploid, with 69 chromosomes instead of 46.

▶ Baun J: *Ob/Gyn Sonography: An Illustrated Review*. Pasadena, CA, Davies Publishing, 2016, pp 36–37.
▶ Sliman MH, Gill KA: The first trimester. In Gill KA: *Ultrasound in Obstetrics and Gynecology: A Practitioner's Guide*. Pasadena, CA, Davies Publishing, 2014, p 185.

651

The postmenarcheal fundal-to-cervical ratio is typically:

a. 2:1–4:1
b. 3:1–4:1
c. 2:1–3:1
d. 3:1–5:1

Gynecology / Normal Pelvic Anatomy

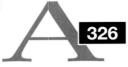

C. 2:1–3:1.

The postmenarcheal nulliparous uterus typically has a fundal-to-cervical ratio of 2:1, while the multiparous uterus has ratio of 3:1.

- Baun J: *Ob/Gyn Sonography: An Illustrated Review*. Pasadena, CA, Davies Publishing, 2016, p 422.
- Raatz Stephenson S (ed): *Diagnostic Medical Sonography: Obstetrics and Gynecology*, 3rd edition. Baltimore, Lippincott Williams & Wilkins, 2012, ch 5.

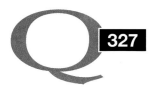

What is the position of the uterus in this transvaginal longitudinal image?

a. anteverted
b. retroverted
c. anteflexed
d. retroflexed

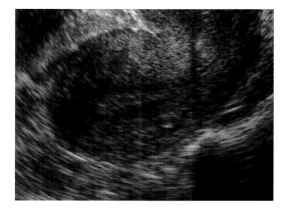

Gynecology / Normal Pelvic Anatomy

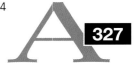

C. Anteflexed.

Transvaginal images are performed with the bladder empty. A normal uterus is anteverted when the bladder is well distended. With the retroflexed/retroverted uterus, the endometrium points toward the right lower corner of the image.

▶ Baun J: *Ob/Gyn Sonography: An Illustrated Review*. Pasadena, CA, Davies Publishing, 2016, pp 352–353.
▶ Gill KA: Gynecology. In Gill KA: *Ultrasound in Obstetrics and Gynecology: A Practitioner's Guide*. Pasadena, CA, Davies Publishing, 2014, pp 36–37.

The best technique for measuring the cervix is:

a. transvaginal
b. transabdominal
c. transperineal
d. translabial

Gynecology / Normal Pelvic Anatomy

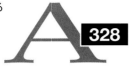

A. Transvaginal.

The most accurate way to measure the cervix is transvaginally. Transabdominal imaging can falsely elongate measurements of the cervix depending on the degree to which the patient's bladder is distended. Overlying bowel gas in the rectum makes it difficult to image the external os using transperineal or translabial technique.

- Baun J: *Ob/Gyn Sonography: An Illustrated Review*. Pasadena, CA, Davies Publishing, 2016, pp 466–467.
- Foy PM: Ultrasound of the cervix during pregnancy. In Gill KA: *Ultrasound in Obstetrics and Gynecology: A Practitioner's Guide*. Pasadena, CA, Davies Publishing, 2014, pp 216–217.

657

This endovaginal image demonstrates the uterus in the longitudinal plane. What is the uterine position?

a. anteflexed
b. retroflexed
c. levoposed
d. dextroposed

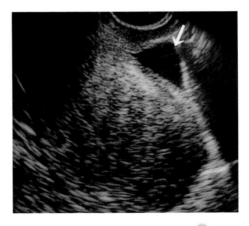

Gynecology / Normal Pelvic Anatomy

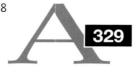

B. Retroflexed.

This image is that of a transvaginal retroflexed uterus, with the uterine fundus pointing to the bottom right of the screen. The levoposed and dextroposed positions are imaged from a transverse/coronal orientation. If the uterus is anteflexed, transvaginally the uterine fundus should point toward the left lower corner of the image.

▶ Baun J: *Ob/Gyn Sonography: An Illustrated Review*. Pasadena, CA, Davies Publishing, 2016, pp 352–353.
▶ Gill KA: Introduction to diagnostic ultrasound. In Gill KA: *Ultrasound in Obstetrics and Gynecology: A Practitioner's Guide*. Pasadena, CA, Davies Publishing, 2014, p 19.

330

Of the following positional terms, which is considered most common uterine position for most women when the urinary bladder is empty?

a. anteverted
b. anteflexed
c. retroverted
d. retroflexed

Gynecology / Normal Pelvic Anatomy

B. Anteflexed.

When the bladder is fully distended, the uterus is anteverted, but most patients do not maintain a fully distended bladder at all times. A retroverted/retroflexed uterus is a backward-tilted uterus.

▶ Baun J: *Ob/Gyn Sonography: An Illustrated Review*. Pasadena, CA, Davies Publishing, 2016, pp 352–353.
▶ Gill KA: Gynecology. In Gill KA: *Ultrasound in Obstetrics and Gynecology: A Practitioner's Guide*. Pasadena, CA, Davies Publishing, 2014, pp 19–20.

Q 331

When one views a sagittal endovaginal image of an anteflexed uterus, the uterine fundus will point to the:

a. right upper corner
b. left lower corner
c. left upper corner
d. right lower corner

Gynecology / Normal Pelvic Anatomy

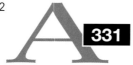

B. Left lower corner.

When imaging the sagittal uterus via endovaginal ultrasound, you will see the uterine fundus of an anteflexed uterus pointing to the lower left corner of the ultrasound screen. The fundus of a retroflexed uterus will point to the lower right corner of the screen.

- Baun J: *Ob/Gyn Sonography: An Illustrated Review*. Pasadena, CA, Davies Publishing, 2016, pp 352–353.
- Gill KA: Introduction to diagnostic ultrasound. In Gill KA: *Ultrasound in Obstetrics and Gynecology: A Practitioner's Guide*. Pasadena, CA, Davies Publishing, 2014, pp 18–20.

The thickness of the endometrium during the proliferative and secretory phases of the menstrual cycle is determined by estrogen and:

a. follicle-stimulating hormone
b. luteinizing hormone
c. estradiol
d. progesterone

Gynecology / Normal Pelvic Anatomy

D. Progesterone.

The fall of estrogen causes sloughing of the endometrial lining, and the rise of estrogen causes the endometrial lining to thicken.

▶ Baun J: *Ob/Gyn Sonography: An Illustrated Review*. Pasadena, CA, Davies Publishing, 2016, pp 350, 363–364.

▶ Hagen-Ansert SL (ed): *Textbook of Diagnostic Ultrasonography*, 7th edition. St. Louis, Elsevier Mosby, 2012, pp 951–952.

333

The distal portion of the cervix:

a. enters the vaginal vault at the level of the fornices
b. lies anterior to the urinary bladder
c. lies anterior to the space of Retzius
d. enters the vaginal vault at the level of the introitus

Gynecology / Normal Pelvic Anatomy

A 333

A. Enters the vaginal vault at the level of the fornices.

The vaginal fornices (singular, *fornix*) are located at the most superior margin of the vagina. The cervix ends at the fornices in the upper vagina. The *introitus* is the exterior opening that leads into the vagina.

▶ Baun J: *Ob/Gyn Sonography: An Illustrated Review*. Pasadena, CA, Davies Publishing, 2016, p 354.
▶ Salem S: Gynecology. In Rumack CM (ed): *Diagnostic Ultrasound*, 4th edition. St. Louis, Mosby, 2011, p 548.

334

The mucosal layer of the uterus is also known as the:

a. zona functionalis
b. zona basalis
c. endometrium
d. myometrium

Gynecology / Normal Pelvic Anatomy

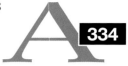

C. Endometrium.

The *endometrium* is the mucosal layer of the uterus. It has a superficial decidual layer called the *zona functionalis* and a basal layer, the *zona basalis*. The basal layer is the permanent layer. The decidual layer is located closer to the cavity of the uterus and is shed monthly with menses.

- Baun J: *Ob/Gyn Sonography: An Illustrated Review*. Pasadena, CA, Davies Publishing, 2016, p 350.
- Callen PW: *Ultrasonography in Obstetrics and Gynecology*, 5th edition. Philadelphia, Elsevier, 2008, pp 909–910.
- Salem S: Gynecology. In Rumack CM (ed): *Diagnostic Ultrasound*, 4th edition. St. Louis, Mosby, 2011, p 552.

 **335**

The uterine corpus–to–cervix ratio in an adult multiparous patient is:

a. 2:1
b. 2:3
c. 2:4
d. 1:2

Gynecology / Normal Pelvic Anatomy

A **335**

A. 2:1.

The corpus (body) of the uterus is approximately twice the length of the cervix in a multiparous woman. In a nulliparous woman the ratio is 1:1.

▶ Baun J: *Ob/Gyn Sonography: An Illustrated Review*. Pasadena, CA, Davies Publishing, 2016, p 422.
▶ Callen PW: *Ultrasonography in Obstetrics and Gynecology*, 5th edition. Philadelphia, Elsevier, 2008, p 909.

Obliteration of the cervix when associated with the process of labor is:

a. funneling
b. effacement
c. engorgement
d. atrophy

Gynecology / Normal Pelvic Anatomy

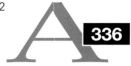

B. Effacement.

From the beginning of labor the cervical canal shortens progressively and a funnel-shaped internal cervical os forms until complete cervical *effacement* is achieved. *Atrophy* suggests a pathologic event. *Engorgement* usually denotes enlargement of ducts or vessels, while *funneling* refers to the bulging of intact membranes within the endocervical canal.

▶ Foy PM: Ultrasound of the cervix during pregnancy. In Gill KA: *Ultrasound in Obstetrics and Gynecology: A Practitioner's Guide*. Pasadena, CA, Davies Publishing, 2014, p 217.

337

The rounded, superior aspect of the uterus located above the insertion of the fallopian tubes is called the:

a. corpus
b. body
c. fundus
d. cornu

Gynecology / Normal Pelvic Anatomy

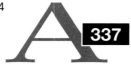

C. Fundus.

The *fundus* is the very top of the uterus, superior to and in between the *cornua* (plural of *cornu*). The cornua are the parts of the uterus to which the fallopian tubes connect. Inferior to the fundus is the body, or *corpus*.

▶ Baun J: *Ob/Gyn Sonography: An Illustrated Review*. Pasadena, CA, Davies Publishing, 2016, pp 349–350.

The thin outer layer of the uterus is the:

a. myometrium
b. serosa
c. endometrium
d. exometrium

Gynecology / Normal Pelvic Anatomy

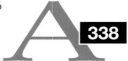

B. Serosa.

The *serosa*, or *perimetrium*, is the outer layer of the uterus. The *myometrium* is the middle, muscular layer, and the *endometrium* is the inner lining.

▶ Baun J: *Ob/Gyn Sonography: An Illustrated Review*. Pasadena, CA, Davies Publishing, 2016, p 350.

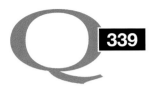

The ovaries always lie in which orientation relative to the broad ligament?

a. lateral
b. medial
c. anterior
d. posterior

Gynecology / Normal Pelvic Anatomy

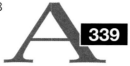

D. Posterior.

The ovaries lie along the posterior border of the broad ligament. The superior border of the broad ligament contains the fallopian tube.

▶ Baun J: *Ob/Gyn Sonography: An Illustrated Review*. Pasadena, CA, Davies Publishing, 2016, pp 349, 356.

Q 340

The outer glandular portion of the ovary that contains the follicles is called the:

a. medulla
b. transitional zone
c. cortex
d. mesovarium

Gynecology / Normal Pelvic Anatomy

C. Cortex.

The ovarian *cortex* is the outer part of the uterus from which follicles emanate. The *medulla* contains the blood vessels. The *mesovarium* is part of the peritoneum, and the *transitional zone* is related to the cervix.

▶ Baun J: *Ob/Gyn Sonography: An Illustrated Review*. Pasadena, CA, Davies Publishing, 2016, pp 356–357.

Q 341

What is the longest portion of the fallopian tube?

a. infundibulum
b. isthmus
c. ampulla
d. interstitial portion

Gynecology / Normal Pelvic Anatomy

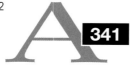

B. Isthmus.

The *isthmus* comprises approximately two-thirds of the fallopian tube's length. The *infundibulum* is the most lateral portion, containing the fimbria, and the *interstitial portion* is closest to the uterus. The *ampulla* is the widened part of the tube where implantation usually occurs.

▶ Baun J: *Ob/Gyn Sonography: An Illustrated Review*. Pasadena, CA, Davies Publishing, 2016, p 356.

The narrowest portion of the fallopian tube that traverses the uterine cornu is called the:

a. isthmic portion
b. ampullary portion
c. interstitial portion
d. infundibulum

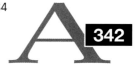

C. Interstitial portion.

The interstitial part of the fallopian tube enters the uterus at the cornu. In order from medial to lateral, the parts of the fallopian tube are the *interstitial portion*, the *isthmus*, the *ampulla*, and the *infundibulum*, from which the lateral-most fimbria project. The interstitial portion is the narrowest part of the tube.

▶ Baun J: *Ob/Gyn Sonography: An Illustrated Review*. Pasadena, CA, Davies Publishing, 2016, p 356.

Which muscle group forms the floor of the pelvis?

a. piriformis
b. levator ani
c. coccygeus
d. iliopsoas

Gynecology / Normal Pelvic Anatomy

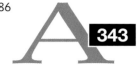

B. Levator ani.

The *levator ani* is formed by three muscles: the coccygeus, pubococcygeus, and iliococcygeus muscles; the puborectalis is part of this group although not usually apparent in sonographic images. The *iliopsoas* are anterior to the iliac wing of the pelvis. The *piriformis* is the triangular muscle located along the lateral wall of the pelvis.

- Baun J: *Ob/Gyn Sonography: An Illustrated Review*. Pasadena, CA, Davies Publishing, 2016, p 347.
- Gill KA: Gynecology. In Gill KA: *Ultrasound in Obstetrics and Gynecology: A Practitioner's Guide*. Pasadena, CA, Davies Publishing, 2014, p 30.

The ligament that provides posterior support to the uterus is the:

a. uterosacral ligament
b. round ligament
c. broad ligament
d. suspensory ligament

Gynecology / Normal Pelvic Anatomy

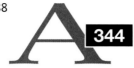

A. Uterosacral ligament.

The *uterosacral*, or *rectouterine*, *ligament* is located on either side of the rectum and connects the uterus to the anterior sacrum. The *suspensory ligament* connects ovary to pelvic wall. The *broad ligament* connects the uterus to the pelvic wall, and the *round ligament* connects the uterus to the upper labia.

▶ Baun J: *Ob/Gyn Sonography: An Illustrated Review*. Pasadena, CA, Davies Publishing, 2016, pp 349, 357.

345

The fibromuscular bands arising from the uterine cornua and extending into the inguinal canal comprise the:

a. broad ligaments
b. uterosacral ligaments
c. round ligaments
d. cardinal ligaments

Gynecology / Normal Pelvic Anatomy

C. Round ligaments.

The round ligaments originate from the uterine cornua near the fallopian tube origins and travel laterally into the inguinal canal, inserting near the top of the labia majora.

Baun J: *Ob/Gyn Sonography: An Illustrated Review*. Pasadena, CA, Davies Publishing, 2016, p 349.

346

The anterior margin of the abdominal and pelvic spaces is formed by the:

a. psoas major
b. obturator internus
c. rectus abdominis
d. piriformis

Gynecology / Normal Pelvic Anatomy

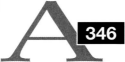

C. Rectus abdominis.

The rectus abdominis muscles are the most anteriorly located. The other muscles are all more posterior. The rectus abdominis muscles are readily evaluated by ultrasound.

▶ Baun J: *Ob/Gyn Sonography: An Illustrated Review*. Pasadena, CA, Davies Publishing, 2016, p 347.

693

What is the name of the double fold of peritoneum that arises from the lateral aspect of the uterus and divides the true pelvis into anterior and posterior compartments?

a. round ligament
b. uterosacral ligament
c. cardinal ligament
d. broad ligament

Gynecology / Normal Pelvic Anatomy

A **347**

D. Broad ligament.

The broad ligament is like a curtain of peritoneum that starts at the uterus and is draped over the fallopian tubes. The broad ligament separates the true pelvis into anterior and posterior compartments.

▶ Baun J: *Ob/Gyn Sonography: An Illustrated Review*. Pasadena, CA, Davies Publishing, 2016, p 349.

695

348

The primary supporting ligament of the uterus arises from the lateral aspect of the cervix and uterus and inserts along the lateral pelvic wall. What is its name?

a. cardinal ligament
b. round ligament
c. broad ligament
d. uterosacral ligament

Gynecology / Normal Pelvic Anatomy

A. 348

A. Cardinal ligament.

The *cardinal ligament* is an extension of the broad ligament, connecting the cervix to the lateral pelvic floor. The *round ligament* connects the uterus to the labia majora, and the *uterosacral ligament* is the posterior part of the cardinal ligament, connecting uterus to sacrum.

▶ Baun J: *Ob/Gyn Sonography: An Illustrated Review*. Pasadena, CA, Davies Publishing, 2016, p 349.
▶ Hagen-Ansert SL (ed): *Textbook of Diagnostic Ultrasonography*, 7th edition. St. Louis, Elsevier Mosby, 2012, pp 945–946.

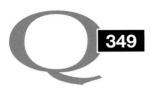

697

The potential space between the anterior abdominal wall and anterior bladder surface is called the:

a. fornix
b. pouch of Douglas
c. cul-de-sac
d. space of Retzius

Gynecology / Normal Pelvic Anatomy

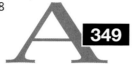

D. Space of Retzius.

The *space of Retzius* lies between the anterior bladder wall and the symphysis pubis. The *fornix* is the space where the superior margin of the vagina encircles the cervix. The *pouch of Douglas* is also known as the *posterior cul-de-sac* and lies between the posterior uterus and the rectum.

▶ Baun J: *Ob/Gyn Sonography: An Illustrated Review*. Pasadena, CA, Davies Publishing, 2016, p 355.

The arrow in this image is pointing toward which cul-de-sac?

a. anterior cul-de-sac
b. space of Retzius
c. Morison's pouch
d. pouch of Douglas

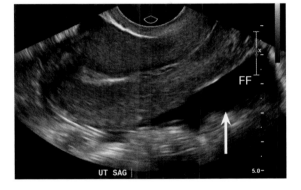

Gynecology / Normal Pelvic Anatomy / AIT—Hotspot

A 350

D. Pouch of Douglas.

The *pouch of Douglas* is the posterior cul-de-sac and a location for free fluid to collect due to its dependent position; this image depicts a small amount of free fluid. The *anterior cul-de-sac* is located between the posterior bladder wall and the anterior uterine surface. *Morison's pouch* is the posterior right subhepatic space. The *space of Retzius* is located between the anterior abdominal wall and the anterior bladder surface.

▶ Baun J: *Ob/Gyn Sonography: An Illustrated Review*. Pasadena, CA, Davies Publishing, 2016, p 355.

351

The space located between the posterior bladder wall and the anterior uterus is called the:

a. anterior cul-de-sac
b. posterior cul-de-sac
c. pouch of Douglas
d. space of Retzius

Gynecology / Normal Pelvic Anatomy

A **351**

A. Anterior cul-de-sac.

The *posterior cul-de-sac* and the *pouch of Douglas* are located between the uterus and the rectum. The *fornix* is around the cervix. The *space of Retzius* lies between the pubic bone and the anterior bladder.

▶ Baun J: *Ob/Gyn Sonography: An Illustrated Review*. Pasadena, CA, Davies Publishing, 2016, p 354.
▶ Gill KA: Gynecology. In Gill KA: *Ultrasound in Obstetrics and Gynecology: A Practitioner's Guide*. Pasadena, CA, Davies Publishing, 2014, pp 31–32.

352

The primary vessels supplying blood to the pelvic organs are the:

a. gonadal arteries
b. spermatic arteries
c. external iliac arteries
d. internal iliac arteries

A 352

D. Internal iliac arteries.

Pelvic organs is a general term referring to all anatomic structures in the pelvic cavity. The *internal iliac arteries* are the trunk arteries that direct blood to all of the pelvic organs, and therefore B is the correct answer. The *gonadal* and *spermatic arteries* are branches of the internal iliac arteries and supply blood to specific structures. The *external iliac artery* supplies blood to the lower extremity.

▶ Baun J: *Ob/Gyn Sonography: An Illustrated Review*. Pasadena, CA, Davies Publishing, 2016, p 358.
▶ Gill KA: *Ultrasound in Obstetrics and Gynecology: A Practitioner's Guide*. Pasadena, CA, Davies Publishing, 2014, p 29.

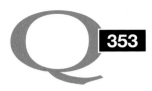

Which arteries penetrate deeply into the myometrium?

a. radial
b. arcuate
c. spiral
d. uterine

Gynecology / Normal Pelvic Anatomy

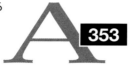

A. Radial.

The radial arteries originate from the peripheral arcuate arteries and penetrate deeply into the myometrium and endometrium. The arcuate arteries also give off the spiral arteries and straight arteries that supply the endometrium.

▶ Hagen-Ansert SL (ed): *Textbook of Diagnostic Ultrasonography*, 7th edition. St. Louis, Elsevier Mosby, 2012, pp 904, 949.

The uterine artery arises from the internal iliac artery and anastomoses with:

a. the external iliac artery
b. a branch of the ovarian artery
c. the common iliac artery
d. the arcuate arteries

Gynecology / Normal Pelvic Anatomy

A 354

B. A branch of the ovarian artery.

The uterine artery gives off the "ovarian branch of the uterine artery," which is commonly assessed with Doppler when evaluation of the ovarian blood supply is desired. The uterine artery is a branch of the internal iliac artery, which comes from the common iliac artery, which arises from the aorta.

▶ Baun J: *Ob/Gyn Sonography: An Illustrated Review*. Pasadena, CA, Davies Publishing, 2016, p 358.

The ovarian artery arises from the:

a. internal iliac artery
b. external iliac artery
c. abdominal aorta
d. vesicular artery

Gynecology / Normal Pelvic Anatomy

A 355

C. Abdominal aorta.

The *ovarian artery* is also called the *gonadal artery*. Both gonadal arteries arise from the abdominal aorta and travel into the pelvis to supply the ovaries with blood. The ovary also receives its blood supply from the ovarian branch of the uterine artery, which anastomoses with the ovarian artery.

▶ Baun J: *Ob/Gyn Sonography: An Illustrated Review*. Pasadena, CA, Davies Publishing, 2016, p 358.

Doppler findings in the ovarian artery supplying the dominant ovary will usually demonstrate:

a. low resistance
b. high resistance
c. high pulsatility
d. low pulsatility

Gynecology / Normal Pelvic Anatomy

A. 356

A. Low resistance.

When there is increased demand for blood flow, such as with an ovary that is producing a follicle, the arteries will dilate, changing the flow to a low-resistance pattern. The increase in arterial lumen diameter, in turn, lowers flow resistance.

▶ Baun J: *Ob/Gyn Sonography: An Illustrated Review*. Pasadena, CA, Davies Publishing, 2016, p 359.

357

Hemodynamic changes occur in the uterine arteries in response to cyclic variations in hormone levels. As the uterus cycles toward menstruation, how do patterns of blood flow change?

a. Uterine artery resistance increases.
b. Uterine artery pulsatility increases.
c. Uterine artery resistance decreases.
d. There is no discernible change in blood flow.

Gynecology / Normal Pelvic Anatomy

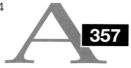

C. Uterine artery resistance decreases.

Decreasing arterial resistance indicates an increase in demand for the oxygen and metabolites carried by blood. As the uterus prepares for the implantation of a conceptus, the endometrium proliferates under the influence of estrogen.

- Baun J: *Ob/Gyn Sonography: An Illustrated Review*. Pasadena, CA, Davies Publishing, 2016, pp 358–359.
- Baun J: Doppler applications in obstetric and gynecologic sonography. In Gill KA: *Ultrasound in Obstetrics and Gynecology: A Practitioner's Guide*. Pasadena, CA, Davies Publishing, 2014, p 385.

358

The resistivity index (RI) is often calculated for quantitative assessment of pelvic organs. Which of the following represents the formula for RI?

a. (peak systolic velocity − end-diastolic velocity) ÷ peak systolic velocity
b. (peak systolic velocity − end-diastolic velocity) ÷ end-diastolic velocity
c. (peak systolic velocity − end-diastolic velocity) ÷ mean velocity
d. (peak systolic velocity − mean velocity) ÷ end-diastolic velocity

Gynecology / Normal Pelvic Anatomy

A 358

A. (peak systolic velocity − end-diastolic velocity) ÷ peak systolic velocity.

The resistivity index (RI) describes downstream resistance to flow, and the higher the resistance to flow, the higher the RI. There are published charts for different organs defining what is normal versus what is abnormal.

▶ Gill KA: Ultrasound in *Obstetrics and Gynecology: A Practitioner's Guide*. Pasadena, CA, Davies Publishing, 2014, p 376.

▶ Raatz Stephenson S (ed): *Diagnostic Medical Sonography: Obstetrics and Gynecology*, 3rd edition. Baltimore, Lippincott Williams & Wilkins, 2012, ch 6.

359

Which of the following is TRUE regarding the performance of transvaginal ultrasound of the pelvis?

a. An empty bladder is preferred for transvaginal examinations.
b. A full bladder is essential for better visualization of the organs.
c. A partially full bladder permits improved visualization of the cervix.
d. A partially full bladder permits improved visualization of the ovaries.

Gynecology / Normal Pelvic Anatomy

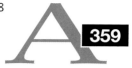

A. An empty bladder is preferred for transvaginal examinations.

For transvaginal ultrasound the patient's bladder should be completely empty. A full or partially full urinary bladder increases patient discomfort and limits visualization due to the relatively small window offered by transvaginal imaging.

- Baun J: *Ob/Gyn Sonography: An Illustrated Review*. Pasadena, CA, Davies Publishing, 2016, p 464.
- Gill KA: Introduction to diagnostic ultrasound. In Gill KA: *Ultrasound in Obstetrics and Gynecology: A Practitioner's Guide*. Pasadena, CA, Davies Publishing, 2014, pp 16, 18.

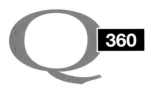

360

Which of the following is TRUE regarding performance of transvaginal ultrasound?

a. If a probe cover is used, high-level disinfection is not needed.
b. Either a sterile probe cover or high-level disinfection must be used.
c. High-level disinfection is always required.
d. The probe does not need to be washed prior to disinfection.

Gynecology / Normal Pelvic Anatomy

A 360

C. High-level disinfection is always required.

High-level disinfection is required after any time an intracavitary probe is used. The probe cover does not need to be sterile as the area of probe insertion is not sterile, although a sterile probe cover may be used for invasive procedures.

▶ Baun J: *Ob/Gyn Sonography: An Illustrated Review*. Pasadena, CA, Davies Publishing, 2016, pp 510–511.

▶ Gill KA: Introduction to diagnostic ultrasound. In Gill KA: *Ultrasound in Obstetrics and Gynecology: A Practitioner's Guide*. Pasadena, CA, Davies Publishing, 2014, pp 16–17, 529–530.

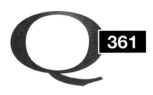

The typical mean diameter of a dominant follicle at ovulation is approximately:

a. 18–20 mm
b. 20–25 mm
c. 16–18 mm
d. 13–14 mm

Gynecology / Physiology

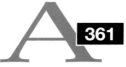

B. 20–25 mm.

The size of the dominant follicle at ovulation is approximately 25 mm.

- Baun J: *Ob/Gyn Sonography: An Illustrated Review*. Pasadena, CA, Davies Publishing, 2016, p 365.
- Gill KA: Gynecology. In Gill KA: Ultrasound in *Obstetrics and Gynecology: A Practitioner's Guide*. Pasadena, CA, Davies Publishing, 2014, p 33.

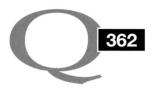

What structure is released from the ovary at ovulation?

a. primary follicle
b. secondary follicle
c. dominant follicle
d. ovum

Gynecology / Physiology

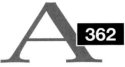

D. Ovum.

The ovum develops inside a part of the follicle called the *cumulus oophorus*. When the follicle ruptures, the ovum is released into the fallopian tube. If the ovum is fertilized, the follicle remnant becomes the *corpus luteum*, which secretes progesterone.

- Baun J: *Ob/Gyn Sonography: An Illustrated Review*. Pasadena, CA, Davies Publishing, 2016, p 365.
- Raatz Stephenson S (ed): *Diagnostic Medical Sonography: Obstetrics and Gynecology*, 3rd edition. Baltimore, Lippincott Williams & Wilkins, 2012, ch 12.

 **363**

Days 1–5 of the ovarian cycle fall within which phase?

a. follicular
b. luteal
c. secretory
d. proliferative

Gynecology / Physiology

A **363**

A. Follicular.

The key term here is *ovarian cycle*. The follicular phase of the ovarian cycle corresponds to the uterine cycle's menstrual (days 1–5) and proliferative (days 6–15) phases. During the follicular stage the follicles grow and a dominant follicle is produced.

▶ Baun J: *Ob/Gyn Sonography: An Illustrated Review*. Pasadena, CA, Davies Publishing, 2016, pp 364–365.
▶ Gill KA: Gynecology. In Gill KA: *Ultrasound in Obstetrics and Gynecology: A Practitioner's Guide*. Pasadena, CA, Davies Publishing, 2014, p 33.

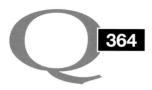

What is the term for the onset of menstruation, usually occurring between 11 and 14 years of age?

a. menopause
b. menarche
c. thelarche
d. pubarche

Gynecology / Physiology

A **364**

B. Menarche.

Menarche is defined as the onset of menstruation. *Menopause* is the end of menstruation. *Thelarche* is defined as breast development as a result of puberty, and *pubarche* is the appearance of pubic hair.

▶ Baun J: *Ob/Gyn Sonography: An Illustrated Review*. Pasadena, CA, Davies Publishing, 2016, p 361.

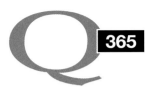

The basis for all current laboratory pregnancy tests is:

a. progesterone
b. beta-hCG
c. estradiol
d. luteinizing hormone

Gynecology / Physiology

A 365

B. Beta-hCG.

Human chorionic gonadotropin (hCG) is a hormone of pregnancy derived from the placental trophoblastic tissue. Measurement of the beta subunit of hCG is the specific test used and may be presented as either quantitative or qualitative results.

▶ Baun J: *Ob/Gyn Sonography: An Illustrated Review*. Pasadena, CA, Davies Publishing, 2016, pp 4–5.

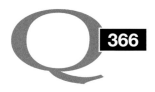

At what rate does hCG increase prior to 8 weeks from the beginning of the last menstrual period?

a. It doubles every month.
b. It doubles every two weeks.
c. It doubles every two days.
d. It doubles daily.

Gynecology / Physiology

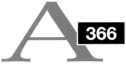

C. It doubles every two days.

Beta-hCG normally doubles every 48–72 hours until 8 weeks after the beginning of the last menstrual period. Thereafter beta-hCG levels off.

▶ Sliman MH, Gill KA: The first trimester. In Gill KA: *Ultrasound in Obstetrics and Gynecology: A Practitioner's Guide.* Pasadena, CA, Davies Publishing, 2014, p 101.

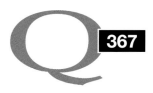

367

If the First International Reference Preparation (FIRP) beta-hCG level is 4000, the Second International Standard (2nd IS) would be approximately:

a. 2000
b. 1000
c. 4000
d. 6000

Gynecology / Physiology

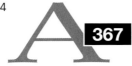

A. 2000.

The Second International Standard is half of the First International Reference Preparation.

- Baun J: *Ob/Gyn Sonography: An Illustrated Review*. Pasadena, CA, Davies Publishing, 2016, p 5.
- Sliman MH, Gill KA: The first trimester. In Gill KA: *Ultrasound in Obstetrics and Gynecology: A Practitioner's Guide*. Pasadena, CA, Davies Publishing, 2014, p 101.

One of the functions of human chorionic gonadotropin is to:

a. stimulate placental growth
b. produce the blastocyst
c. produce the zygote
d. support the corpus luteum

Gynecology / Physiology

A **368**

D. Support the corpus luteum.

The release of human chorionic gonadotropin (hCG) signals the corpus luteum to remain active and produce progesterone to support the pregnancy. Without hCG, the corpus luteum involutes and the menstrual cycle continues.

▶ Baun J: *Ob/Gyn Sonography: An Illustrated Review*. Pasadena, CA, Davies Publishing, 2016, pp 4–5.

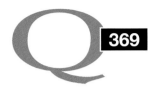

High serum levels of beta-hCG can suggest:

a. anembryonic pregnancy
b. ectopic pregnancy
c. multiple pregnancy
d. impending abortion

Gynecology / Physiology

A 369

C. Multiple pregnancy.

Of the choices listed, multiple pregnancy is the best answer. The other choices would show low or decreasing levels of beta-hCG. In addition to multiple pregnancies, elevated beta-hCG titers may indicate the presence of gestational trophoblastic disease.

▶ Baun J: *Ob/Gyn Sonography: An Illustrated Review*. Pasadena, CA, Davies Publishing, 2016, pp 4–5, 274.
▶ Sliman MH, Gill KA: The first trimester. In Gill KA: *Ultrasound in Obstetrics and Gynecology: A Practitioner's Guide*. Pasadena, CA, Davies Publishing, 2014, pp 101–102.

Human chorionic gonadotropin is actively secreted by:

a. trophoblastic tissue
b. ovaries
c. pituitary gland
d. adrenal gland

Gynecology / Physiology

A 370

A. Trophoblastic tissue.

The trophoblastic tissue of the blastocyst is responsible for secreting beta-hCG. It is the trophoblast that becomes the placenta. The organs listed in the other choices do not secrete beta-hCG.

▶ Baun J: *Ob/Gyn Sonography: An Illustrated Review*. Pasadena, CA, Davies Publishing, 2016, p 4.

The outermost layer of the follicular cells surrounding the ovum is called the:

a. zona pellucida
b. corona radiata
c. nucleus
d. plasma membrane

Gynecology / Physiology

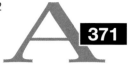

B. Corona radiata.

The *corona radiata* is the outer layer of the ovum, comprising follicular cells. Sperm must penetrate this tough outer layer in order to fertilize the egg. The layer located more centrally but next to the corona radiata is the *zona pellucida*.

- Baun J: *Ob/Gyn Sonography: An Illustrated Review*. Pasadena, CA, Davies Publishing, 2016, p 6.
- Raatz Stephenson S (ed): *Diagnostic Medical Sonography: Obstetrics and Gynecology*, 3rd edition. Baltimore, Lippincott Williams & Wilkins, 2012, ch 13.

Q 372

Fertilization usually occurs in which portion of the fallopian tube?

a. interstitial
b. ampullary
c. cornual
d. fimbrial

Gynecology / Physiology

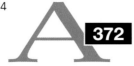

B. Ampullary.

Normal fertilization occurs in the lateral one-third or ampullary portion of the fallopian tube. Fertilization in the other areas listed could result in an ectopic pregnancy.

- Baun J: *Ob/Gyn Sonography: An Illustrated Review*. Pasadena, CA, Davies Publishing, 2016, pp 6, 355.
- Sliman MH, Gill KA: The first trimester. In Gill KA: *Ultrasound in Obstetrics and Gynecology: A Practitioner's Guide*. Pasadena, CA, Davies Publishing, 2014, p 90.

745

What is the name of the structure that surrounds the ovum as it is extruded from the follicle on approximately menstrual day 14?

a. corpus albicans
b. cumulus oophorus
c. zona basalis
d. zona pellucida

Gynecology / Physiology

A **373**

D. Zona pellucida.

The *zona pellucida* consists of a layer of glycoprotein cells that lies interior to the corona radiata and is responsible for ensuring that only one sperm fertilizes the egg. The zona pellucida remains until implantation, after which it degenerates.

▶ Baun J: *Ob/Gyn Sonography: An Illustrated Review*. Pasadena, CA, Davies Publishing, 2016, p 6.
▶ Moore KL, Persaud TVN, Torchia MG: *The Developing Human: Clinically Oriented Embryology*, 9th edition. Philadelphia, Elsevier Saunders, 2013, pp 18–19.

Q 374

The male germ cells are the:

a. spermatozoa
b. Leydig cells
c. testes
d. androgens

Gynecology / Physiology

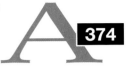

A. Spermatozoa.

Spermatozoa are the male germ cells, or *gametes*. The female gamete is the *ovum*. Gametes are haploid, meaning that they contain half the full complement of chromosomes; a sperm cell contains 22 chromosomes plus either an X or a Y (sex) chromosome. At fertilization, a single sperm cell combines with the ovum (which contains 22 chromosomes plus an X chromosome) to create the earliest form of the conceptus, the *zygote*.

- Baun J: *Ob/Gyn Sonography: An Illustrated Review*. Pasadena, CA, Davies Publishing, 2016, p 6.
- Moore KL, Persaud TVN, Torchia MG: *The Developing Human: Clinically Oriented Embryology*, 9th edition. Philadelphia, Elsevier Saunders, 2013, p 19.

375

When fertilization does NOT occur, the corpus luteum regresses into the:

a. primary follicle
b. secondary follicle
c. Graafian follicle
d. corpus albicans

Gynecology / Physiology

A 375

D. Corpus albicans.

After the corpus luteum regresses into the corpus albicans, estrogen and progesterone decrease.

▶ Baun J: *Ob/Gyn Sonography: An Illustrated Review*. Pasadena, CA, Davies Publishing, 2016, p 364.

▶ Raatz Stephenson S (ed): *Diagnostic Medical Sonography: Obstetrics and Gynecology*, 3rd edition. Baltimore, Lippincott Williams & Wilkins, 2012, ch 4.

376

Fertilization occurs approximately how soon after ovulation?

a. 12–24 hours
b. 24–36 hours
c. 3–5 days
d. 7–10 days

Gynecology / Physiology

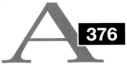

A. 12–24 hours.

After the ovum is released from the ovary, it waits in the fallopian tube up to 24 hours for fertilization to occur. If fertilization does not occur, the ovum dies.

▶ Baun J: *Ob/Gyn Sonography: An Illustrated Review*. Pasadena, CA, Davies Publishing, 2016, p 5.
▶ Sliman MH, Gill KA: The first trimester. In Gill KA: *Ultrasound in Obstetrics and Gynecology: A Practitioner's Guide*. Pasadena, CA, Davies Publishing, 2014, p 90.

This image was obtained from a patient undergoing infertility treatment. Which of the following can be inferred based solely on this image?

a. Ovulation has already occurred.
b. Ovulation will occur within 36 hours.
c. Hormonal therapy has failed.
d. An ectopic pregnancy has implanted on the ovary.

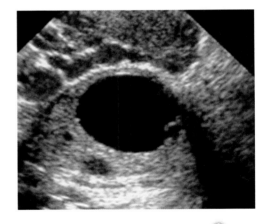

Gynecology / Physiology / AIT—PACSim

A **377**

B. Ovulation will occur within 36 hours.

The cystic structure adjacent to the wall of this dominant follicle is the cumulus oophorus. Once the cumulus oophorus can be visualized, ovulation usually occurs within 36 hours.

▶ Baun J: *Ob/Gyn Sonography: An Illustrated Review*. Pasadena, CA, Davies Publishing, 2016, pp 364–365.

Which of the following is a feminizing tumor that may lead to precocious puberty?

a. teratoma
b. serous cystadenoma
c. granulosa cell tumor
d. arrhenoblastoma

Gynecology / Pediatric

A 378

C. Granulosa cell tumor.

Granulosa cell tumors, also known as *theca cell tumors*, occur prepubertally in 5% of cases and are typically unilateral with bilateral involvement less than 5% of the time. These tumors can exhibit late recurrence and may present as precocious puberty.

▶ Baun J: *Ob/Gyn Sonography: An Illustrated Review*. Pasadena, CA, Davies Publishing, 2016, p 395.

▶ Martin J, Woolpert L, Raatz Stephenson S: Pediatric pelvis. In Raatz Stephenson S (ed): *Diagnostic Medical Sonography: Obstetrics and Gynecology*, 3rd edition. Philadelphia, Lippincott Williams & Wilkins, 2012, ch 7.

The cause of central precocious puberty is:

a. excessive estrogen levels
b. related to a tumor of the ovary at birth
c. excessive progesterone levels
d. activation of the hypothalamic-pituitary-gonadal axis

Gynecology / Pediatric

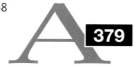

D. Activation of the hypothalamic-pituitary-gonadal axis.

Central precocious puberty may occur as a result of a central nervous system problem, such as a tumor, but it is usually idiopathic. *Peripheral precocious puberty* is a result of a problem with estrogen or a pelvic tumor.

- Baun J: *Ob/Gyn Sonography: An Illustrated Review*. Pasadena, CA, Davies Publishing, 2016, p 427.
- Martin J, Woolpert L, Raatz Stephenson S: Pediatric pelvis. In Raatz Stephenson S (ed): *Diagnostic Medical Sonography: Obstetrics and Gynecology*, 3rd edition. Philadelphia, Lippincott Williams & Wilkins, 2012, ch 7.

Q 380

An accumulation of fluid in the vagina but not the uterus of a premenarcheal patient is called:

a. hydrocolpos
b. hematometrocolpos
c. hematometra
d. hydrometra

Gynecology / Pediatric

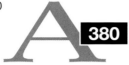

A. Hydrocolpos.

The prefix *hydro* means fluid, and *colpos* means vagina. Therefore, *hydrocolpos* is fluid in the vagina. *Hemato* means blood, and *metra/metro* refers to the uterus. Therefore, *hematometrocolpos* means blood in the uterus and vagina, *hematometra* means blood in the uterus, and *hydrometra* means fluid in the uterus.

▶ Martin J, Woolpert L, Raatz Stephenson S: Pediatric pelvis. In Raatz Stephenson S (ed): *Diagnostic Medical Sonography: Obstetrics and Gynecology*, 3rd edition. Philadelphia, Lippincott Williams & Wilkins, 2012, ch 7.

The most common cause of hematocolpos is:

a. vaginal agenesis
b. bladder-vaginal fistula
c. acquired gynatresia
d. imperforate hymen

Gynecology / Pediatric

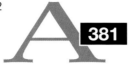

D. Imperforate hymen.

The most common cause of hematocolpos, which is menstrual blood in the vaginal canal, is an imperforate hymen. The other choices are uncommon causes. Hydrocolpos, hematometra, and hydrometra are also typically due to an imperforate hymen. (See the answer to question 380.)

- Baun J: *Ob/Gyn Sonography: An Illustrated Review*. Pasadena, CA, Davies Publishing, 2016, p 425.
- Gill KA: Gynecology. In Gill KA: *Ultrasound in Obstetrics and Gynecology: A Practitioner's Guide*. Pasadena, CA, Davies Publishing, 2014, p 42.

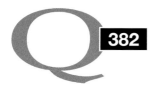

A 14-year-old girl presents with a palpable midline pelvic mass and amenorrhea. A sagittal ultrasound section through a full bladder yields the accompanying image. The most likely diagnosis is:

a. sarcoma botryoides
b. hydrometrocolpos
c. uterine tumor
d. vaginal rhabdomyosarcoma

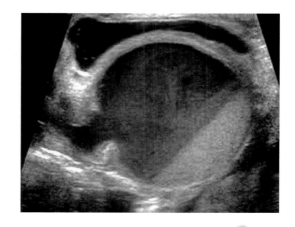

Gynecology / Pediatric / AIT—PACSim

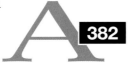

B. Hydrometrocolpos.

In a 14-year-old girl with amenorrhea and the findings presented in this image, the most likely diagnosis is hematometrocolpos, blood in the uterus and vagina; hence the best answer is *hydrometrocolpos* (which refers generally to fluid in the uterus and vagina). Notice the fluid-fluid level from the standing blood and the partially full bladder superficially. The other choices are less likely, given the ultrasound findings and this patient's clinical history.

▶ Baun J: *Ob/Gyn Sonography: An Illustrated Review*. Pasadena, CA, Davies Publishing, 2016, pp 372, 423–425.

Androgenic tumors, such as Sertoli-Leydig cell tumors, cause:

a. precocious puberty
b. fibrocystic breasts
c. hirsutism
d. postmenopausal bleeding

Gynecology / Pediatric

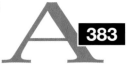

C. Hirsutism.

Androgenic tumors secrete testosterone and cause masculinization. Also called *androblastomas*, these uncommon benign tumors account for less than 0.5% of all ovarian tumors and typically present in the second to third decade of life. About half of patients demonstrate clinical signs of androgenic hormone production such as oligomenorrhea that may proceed into amenorrhea, hirsutism, hoarseness, and breast atrophy. All of the other symptoms would arise from estrogenic sources.

- Baun J: *Ob/Gyn Sonography: An Illustrated Review*. Pasadena, CA, Davies Publishing, 2016, p 396.
- Gill KA: Gynecology. In Gill KA: *Ultrasound in Obstetrics and Gynecology: A Practitioner's Guide*. Pasadena, CA, Davies Publishing, 2014, pp 70, 71.

Female pseudohermaphroditism may be caused by:

a. DES exposure
b. congenital adrenal hyperplasia
c. decreased progesterone production
d. decreased androgens

Gynecology / Pediatric

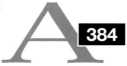

B. Congenital adrenal hyperplasia.

A female pseudohermaphrodite has a 46,XX karyotype and has ovaries but masculinized external genitalia. This condition can also be caused by an increased production of androgens.

▶ Baun J: *Ob/Gyn Sonography: An Illustrated Review*. Pasadena, CA, Davies Publishing, 2016, p 427.
▶ Martin J, Woolpert L, Raatz Stephenson S: Pediatric pelvis. In Raatz Stephenson S (ed): *Diagnostic Medical Sonography: Obstetrics and Gynecology*, 3rd edition. Philadelphia, Lippincott Williams & Wilkins, 2012, ch 7.

385

Which of the following is correct regarding true hermaphroditism?

a. The genitalia are visibly male but there are ovaries.
b. There is ambiguous genitalia and male or female gonads.
c. There is a mosaicism with both male and female gonadal cells.
d. The genitalia are visibly female but there are testicles in the abdomen.

Gynecology / Pediatric

A 385

C. There is a mosaicism with both male and female gonadal cells.

In a true hermaphrodite the cells are usually mosaic for XX and XY and there are components of both ovaries and testicles. True hermaphroditism is rare in humans.

▶ Baun J: *Ob/Gyn Sonography: An Illustrated Review*. Pasadena, CA, Davies Publishing, 2016, p 427.

▶ Raatz Stephenson S (ed): *Diagnostic Medical Sonography: Obstetrics and Gynecology*, 3rd edition. Baltimore, Lippincott Williams & Wilkins, 2012, ch 7.

A 24-year-old patient presents externally as a female, but chromosome analysis reveals a 46,XY karyotype. What looks like intra-abdominal ovaries are actually testicles, and the uterus is absent. This patient most likely has what condition?

a. testicular feminization
b. true hermaphroditism
c. congenital adrenal hyperplasia
d. androgenic tumor

Gynecology / Pediatric / AIT—PACSim

A. Testicular feminization.

Testicular feminization, or *androgen insensitivity syndrome*, presents with female external characteristics but with 46,XY chromosomes and either testicles or one testicle and a streak gonad. *True hermaphrodites* have both female and male gonadal tissue. *Androgenic tumors* and *congenital adrenal hyperplasia* (CAH) cause masculinization of an otherwise normal female.

▶ Baun J: *Ob/Gyn Sonography: An Illustrated Review*. Pasadena, CA, Davies Publishing, 2016, p 427.

▶ Raatz Stephenson S (ed): *Diagnostic Medical Sonography: Obstetrics and Gynecology*, 3rd edition. Baltimore, Lippincott Williams & Wilkins, 2012, ch 7.

What is the normal volume of a neonatal ovary?

a. ≤1.0 cc
b. ≥1.0 cc
c. 2–3 cc
d. 3–4 cc

Gynecology / Pediatric

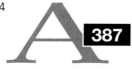

B. ≥1.0 cc.

The normal neonatal ovarian volume is approximately 1.0 cc or greater.

▶ Baun J: *Ob/Gyn Sonography: An Illustrated Review*. Pasadena, CA, Davies Publishing, 2016, pp 346, 423.

388

In a premenarcheal 5-year-old, what is the fundal-to-cervical ratio?

a. 1:3
b. 1:1
c. 3:1
d. 2:1

Gynecology / Pediatric

A 388

B. 1:1.

The fundal-to-cervical ratio in the prepubescent child is 1:1. At puberty the ratio is 2:1 until the patient is multiparous, at which point the ratio is 3:1. In postmenopausal women the ratio is 1:1 again.

▶ Baun J: *Ob/Gyn Sonography: An Illustrated Review*. Pasadena, CA, Davies Publishing, 2016, p 422.

▶ Raatz Stephenson S (ed): *Diagnostic Medical Sonography: Obstetrics and Gynecology*, 3rd edition. Baltimore, Lippincott Williams & Wilkins, 2012, ch 5.

In these images, what structure of interest is visualized in the intrauterine area?

a. endometrial fluid
b. leiomyoma
c. intrauterine contraceptive device
d. adenomyosis

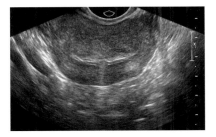

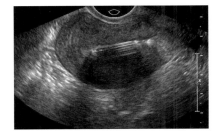

Gynecology / Infertility and Endocrinology

A **389**

C. Intrauterine contraceptive device.

This patient has a Mirena IUCD. In the transverse plane (top image), the echogenic arms of the device are clearly visible. In the sagittal plane (bottom image), there is the classic IUCD appearance of parallel echogenic lines with artifactual shadowing.

▶ Baun J: *Ob/Gyn Sonography: An Illustrated Review*. Pasadena, CA, Davies Publishing, 2016, pp 412–413.

▶ Gill KA: Gynecology. In Gill KA: *Ultrasound in Obstetrics and Gynecology: A Practitioner's Guide*. Pasadena, CA, Davies Publishing, 2014, pp 74–76.

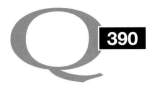

This patient is a 27-year-old seeing her physician to check the placement of her intrauterine device placement. What findings are evident in this image?

a. No IUD is present within the uterus.
b. The IUD is in the normal location.
c. The IUD is located too inferiorly.
d. The IUD has perforated the uterine fundus.

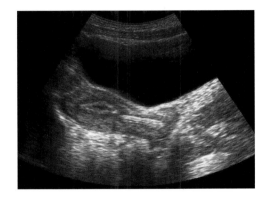

Gynecology / Infertility and Endocrinology / AIT—PACSim

A **390**

C. The IUD is located too inferiorly.

The image demonstrates that the IUD has slipped out of the uterine fundus and is inferiorly located in the cervix. A small amount of free fluid is located in the endometrial canal. Note that the terms *IUD* (intrauterine device) and *IUCD* (intrauterine contraceptive device) are often used interchangeably.

▶ Baun J: *Ob/Gyn Sonography: An Illustrated Review*. Pasadena, CA, Davies Publishing, 2016, pp 412–413.

▶ Gill KA: Gynecology. In Gill KA: *Ultrasound in Obstetrics and Gynecology: A Practitioner's Guide*. Pasadena, CA, Davies Publishing, 2014, pp 74–76.

The most common cause of male infertility is:

a. cryptorchidism
b. varicoceles
c. testicular failure
d. spermatic cord obstruction

Gynecology / Infertility and Endocrinology

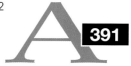

B. Varicoceles.

Varicoceles are dilated veins in the scrotum surrounding the testicle. Dilated veins increase the temperature and destroy the spermatozoa. All the choices can be causes of male infertility, but the varicocele is the most common and is correctable.

- Baun J: *Ob/Gyn Sonography: An Illustrated Review*. Pasadena, CA, Davies Publishing, 2016, p 410.
- Koulianos G, Gill KA: Infertility. In Gill KA: *Ultrasound in Obstetrics and Gynecology: A Practitioner's Guide*. Pasadena, CA, Davies Publishing, 2014, p 393.

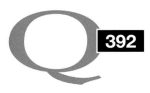

Adhesions within the endometrial cavity are referred to as:

a. polyps
b. mucosa
c. synechiae
d. adenomyosis

Gynecology / Infertility and Endocrinology

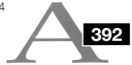

C. Synechiae.

Synechiae are adhesions found within the endometrial cavity, usually seen only in the presence of fluid within the endometrial cavity, such as with a pregnancy or on hysterosonography. Adhesions may be caused by surgical manipulation of the endometrium, as occurs with dilatation and curettage (D&C).

- Baun J: *Ob/Gyn Sonography: An Illustrated Review*. Pasadena, CA, Davies Publishing, 2016, p 375.
- Koulianos G, Gill KA: Infertility. In Gill KA: *Ultrasound in Obstetrics and Gynecology: A Practitioner's Guide*. Pasadena, CA, Davies Publishing, 2014, p 400.

When a radiopaque dye is introduced into the uterus and fallopian tubes for visualization on x-rays, the procedure is called:

a. sonohysterography
b. laparoscopy
c. hysterography
d. endoscopy

Gynecology / Infertility and Endocrinology

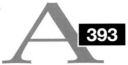

C. Hysterography.

The key phrase here is "visualization on x-rays." *Hysterography* is radiography performed using a small camera at the end of a tube that is placed inside the uterus through a small incision. This exam is also called *hysterosalpingography* (HSG) because the contrast can be seen going through the fallopian tubes, performed sometimes for infertility. *Sonohysterography* is the ultrasound version of imaging the uterine cavity by introducing fluid into the cavity and capturing images with ultrasound. *Laparoscopy* uses a small camera at the end of a tube that is placed through a small incision in the abdomen. *Endoscopy* uses a small camera at the end of a catheter placed in the rectum or esophagus for viewing.

▶ Baun J: Doppler applications in obstetric and gynecologic sonography. In Gill KA: *Ultrasound in Obstetrics and Gynecology: A Practitioner's Guide*. Pasadena, CA, Davies Publishing, 2014, pp 415, 419, 501–504.

▶ Koulianos G, Gill KA: Infertility. In Gill KA: *Ultrasound in Obstetrics and Gynecology: A Practitioner's Guide*. Pasadena, CA, Davies Publishing, 2014, pp 400–401.

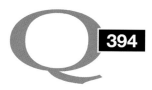

Which of the following is NOT used to treat infertility patients?

a. clomiphene citrate
b. human chorionic gonadotropin
c. metformin
d. methotrexate

Gynecology / Infertility and Endocrinology

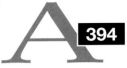

D. Methotrexate.

Methotrexate is an antifolate drug that inhibits cell division and has been used not only as chemotherapy for cancer patients but also to treat ectopic pregnancy and gestational trophoblastic disease in ob/gyn patients. The other drugs are all used to treat infertility. Although most familiar as an antidiabetic drug, metformin (Glucophage) may be used to induce ovulation because of the relationship between elevated insulin levels and insulin resistance.

- Baun J: *Ob/Gyn Sonography: An Illustrated Review*. Pasadena, CA, Davies Publishing, 2016, pp 413–414.
- Gill KA: *Ultrasound in Obstetrics and Gynecology: A Practitioner's Guide*. Pasadena, CA, Davies Publishing, 2014, pp 59, 110, 199, 222, 397.

395

For which of the disorders below might a patient with infertility be prescribed heparin?

a. endometriosis
b. theca-lutein cysts
c. fibroids
d. factor V Leiden

A 395

D. Factor V Leiden.

Factor V Leiden (pronounced "factor five LI-den") is a blood-clotting disorder that causes excessive clotting, which can lead to infertility and other problems in pregnancy. Heparin may be prescribed to prevent the clots from forming. Coumadin, another anticlotting drug, cannot be used in pregnancy because it is associated with a severe risk of fetal malformation.

▶ Cunningham FG, Leveno KJ, Bloom SL, et al: *Williams Obstetrics*, 24th edition. New York, McGraw-Hill, 2014, pp 1031–1032.

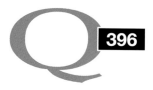

Which of the following is a disorder resulting from physiologic sensitivity to gonadotropins?

a. polycystic ovarian disease
b. luteinized unruptured follicle syndrome
c. ovarian hyperstimulation syndrome
d. endometrioma

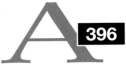

C. Ovarian hyperstimulation syndrome.

Ovarian hyperstimulation syndrome occurs as a response to infertility treatment involving clomiphene or gonadotropins, although it is more likely to occur with gonadotropin treatment. Ovarian hyperstimulation can range from mild to severe.

▶ Baun J: *Ob/Gyn Sonography: An Illustrated Review*. Pasadena, CA, Davies Publishing, 2016, p 414.
▶ Raatz Stephenson S (ed): *Diagnostic Medical Sonography: Obstetrics and Gynecology*, 3rd edition. Baltimore, Lippincott Williams & Wilkins, 2012, ch 12.
▶ Wiseman DA, Greene CA, Pierson RA: Infertility. In Rumack CM (ed): *Diagnostic Ultrasound*. St. Louis, Mosby, 1998, pp 1407–1439.

If human menopausal gonadotropin (hMG) leads to successful follicular development, the fertility specialist then administers:

a. estrogen
b. human chorionic gonadotropin
c. follicle-stimulating hormone
d. luteinizing hormone

Gynecology / Infertility and Endocrinology

A 397

B. Human chorionic gonadotropin.

Human menopausal gonadotropin (hMG) contains both luteinizing hormone and follicle-stimulating hormone. After administration of hMG and successful follicular development, human chorionic gonadotropin (hCG) is typically administered to induce ovulation.

▶ Baun J: *Ob/Gyn Sonography: An Illustrated Review*. Pasadena, CA, Davies Publishing, 2016, p 410.

In an infertility patient, when can the dominant ovarian follicle be identified sonographically?

a. days 3–5
b. days 5–7
c. days 7–9
d. days 9–10

Gynecology / Infertility and Endocrinology

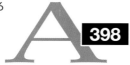

B. Days 5–7.

Follicles start out at about 5–6 mm in diameter and grow approximately 2 mm per day. Between days 5 and 7, one becomes dominant and is visible by transvaginal ultrasound.

- Baun J: *Ob/Gyn Sonography: An Illustrated Review*. Pasadena, CA, Davies Publishing, 2016, p 416.
- Koulianos G, Gill KA: Infertility. In Gill KA: *Ultrasound in Obstetrics and Gynecology: A Practitioner's Guide*. Pasadena, CA, Davies Publishing, 2014, p 395.

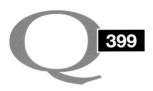

The abbreviation that refers to placing an egg into the fallopian tube after it has been fertilized in a Petri dish is:

a. ART
b. GIFT
c. ZIFT
d. IVF

Gynecology / Infertility and Endocrinology

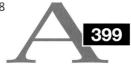

C. ZIFT.

Although both GIFT and ZIFT involve placing the egg into the fallopian tube, only in ZIFT is the egg first fertilized in the Petri dish. *ZIFT* stands for *zygote intrafallopian transfer*; a zygote is a fertilized egg. *ART* stands for *assisted reproductive technology* (a broad term encompassing all types of infertility treatment), *GIFT* for *gamete intrafallopian transfer*, and *IVF* for *in vitro fertilization*.

▶ Baun J: *Ob/Gyn Sonography: An Illustrated Review*. Pasadena, CA, Davies Publishing, 2016, p 415.
▶ Koulianos G, Gill KA: Infertility. In Gill KA: *Ultrasound in Obstetrics and Gynecology: A Practitioner's Guide*. Pasadena, CA, Davies Publishing, 2014, p 402.

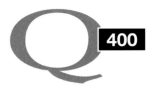

400

What is the type of infertility treatment in which the ovaries are stimulated and then ova are retrieved and mixed with sperm outside the uterus?

a. IVF
b. GIFT
c. ZIFT
d. embryo transfer

Gynecology / Infertility and Endocrinology

A 400

A. IVF.

With in vitro fertilization (IVF), ova are retrieved following ovarian stimulation. The ova are mixed with sperm in a Petri dish. Embryos are formed and then implanted into the uterus with embryo transfer. ZIFT and GIFT are not as common. See also the answer to question 399.

▶ Baun J: *Ob/Gyn Sonography: An Illustrated Review*. Pasadena, CA, Davies Publishing, 2016, pp 414–415.

▶ Koulianos G, Gill KA: Infertility. In Gill KA: *Ultrasound in Obstetrics and Gynecology: A Practitioner's Guide*. Pasadena, CA, Davies Publishing, 2014, pp 402–403.

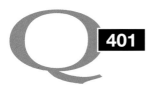

What is the normal appearance of the postmenopausal endometrium?

a. thick and homogeneously echogenic
b. thin and homogeneously echogenic
c. hypoechoic and thicker than 8 mm
d. thin and heterogeneous

Gynecology / Postmenopausal

A **401**

B. Thin and homogeneously echogenic.

The normal postmenopausal endometrium in a patient not on hormone replacement is thin, echogenic, and homogeneous.

▶ Baun J: *Ob/Gyn Sonography: An Illustrated Review*. Pasadena, CA, Davies Publishing, 2016, p 428.

▶ Gill KA: Gynecology. In Gill KA: *Ultrasound in Obstetrics and Gynecology: A Practitioner's Guide*. Pasadena, CA, Davies Publishing, 2014, pp 26–27, 34–35.

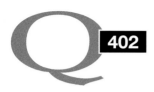

803

Which double-thickness measurement of the postmenopausal endometrium is generally accepted to be normal?

a. 5–7 mm
b. 6–8 mm
c. <5 mm
d. >5 mm

Gynecology / Postmenopausal

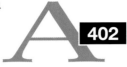

C. <5 mm.

Postmenopausally, the endometrium should measure less than 5 mm. If the patient is on hormone therapy or receiving treatments such as tamoxifen, the endometrium may be thicker.

▶ Baun J: *Ob/Gyn Sonography: An Illustrated Review*. Pasadena, CA, Davies Publishing, 2016, p 428.

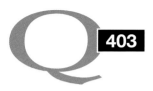

In the absence of hormonal stimulation, what is the normal course of the postmenopausal ovaries?

a. They decrease in size.
b. They increase in size but extrude fewer follicles.
c. They stay the same size.
d. They stay the same size but extrude fewer follicles.

Gynecology / Postmenopausal

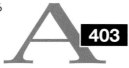

A. They decrease in size.

The postmenopausal ovaries decrease in size with age to the point where they may be impossible to visualize with ultrasound.

- Baun J: *Ob/Gyn Sonography: An Illustrated Review*. Pasadena, CA, Davies Publishing, 2016, p 428.
- Raatz Stephenson S (ed): *Diagnostic Medical Sonography: Obstetrics and Gynecology*, 3rd edition. Baltimore, Lippincott Williams & Wilkins, 2012, ch 4.

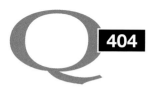

Which of the following is a side effect of decreased hormonal production during menopause?

a. increased irregular bleeding
b. enlargement of fibroids
c. breast enlargement
d. decreased cervical mucus

Gynecology / Postmenopausal

A 404

D. Decreased cervical mucus.

Decreased hormone production causes several physiologic changes in the postmenopausal body. One of these changes is decreased cervical mucus.

▶ Raatz Stephenson S (ed): *Diagnostic Medical Sonography: Obstetrics and Gynecology*, 3rd edition. Baltimore, Lippincott Williams & Wilkins, 2012, ch 4.

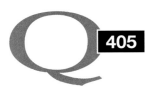

Which pharmaceutical agent commonly used to treat estrogen-sensitive types of breast cancer may alter the typical appearance of the endometrium?

a. clomiphene citrate (Clomid)
b. menotropin (Pergonal)
c. methotrexate
d. tamoxifen

Gynecology / Postmenopausal

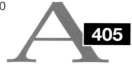

D. Tamoxifen.

Tamoxifen is an antiestrogenic drug commonly used in patients with breast cancer. It may cause endometrial hyperplasia or cancer, and therefore the endometria of women taking tamoxifen are routinely evaluated with transvaginal sonography.

▶ Baun J: *Ob/Gyn Sonography: An Illustrated Review*. Pasadena, CA, Davies Publishing, 2016, pp 429, 430.

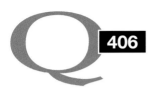

Postmenopausal patients receiving unopposed estrogen as hormone replacement therapy may exhibit a normal endometrial thickness of up to:

a. 5 mm
b. 8 mm
c. 6 mm
d. 7 mm

Gynecology / Postmenopausal

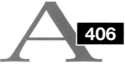

A 406

B. 8 mm.

In a postmenopausal patient on estrogen-replacement therapy, the endometrium may measure up to 8 mm. An endometrial thickness greater than 8 mm is cause for concern and should be further investigated.

▶ Baun J: *Ob/Gyn Sonography: An Illustrated Review*. Pasadena, CA, Davies Publishing, 2016, p 429.

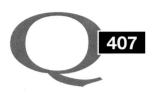

407

The primary clinical symptom in patients with endometrial carcinoma is:

a. pain
b. polyuria
c. vaginal bleeding
d. menorrhagia

Gynecology / Postmenopausal

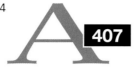

C. Vaginal bleeding.

Vaginal bleeding as a symptom of endometrial carcinoma is more typically seen in postmenopausal patients. Although not all postmenopausal bleeding is due to cancer, any postmenopausal patient with vaginal bleeding must undergo a full workup and possibly endometrial biopsy to rule out endometrial cancer.

▶ Baun J: *Ob/Gyn Sonography: An Illustrated Review*. Pasadena, CA, Davies Publishing, 2016, pp 381–383.
▶ Gill KA: Gynecology. In Gill KA: *Ultrasound in Obstetrics and Gynecology: A Practitioner's Guide*. Pasadena, CA, Davies Publishing, 2014, p 52.

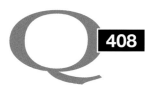

A biochemical marker that can be elevated in cases of ovarian carcinoma is:

a. PAP
b. CA-125
c. MSAFP
d. SAP

Gynecology / Postmenopausal

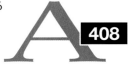

B. CA-125.

CA-125 is a marker for ovarian cancer, although most ovarian cancer is still found after it has metastasized. CA-125 is not specific to ovarian cancer and may be found in the presence of other pathologies as well. According to the American Cancer Society, age greater than 50 is one of the major risk factors for ovarian cancer, and half of all ovarian cancers are found in women 63 years of age and older.

- Baun J: *Ob/Gyn Sonography: An Illustrated Review*. Pasadena, CA, Davies Publishing, 2016, p 390.
- Gill KA: Gynecology. In Gill KA: *Ultrasound in Obstetrics and Gynecology: A Practitioner's Guide*. Pasadena, CA, Davies Publishing, 2014, p 72.

Q 409

Endometrial polyps are more easily seen and best demonstrated by:

a. laparoscopy
b. transvaginal sonography
c. full-bladder transabdominal sonography
d. hysterosonography

Gynecology / Postmenopausal

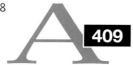

D. Hysterosonography.

Hysterosonography (or *sonohysterography*) involves instilling fluid into the endometrial canal and performing transvaginal ultrasound to visualize the endometrium. Polyps are well visualized with this technique.

- Baun J: *Ob/Gyn Sonography: An Illustrated Review*. Pasadena, CA, Davies Publishing, 2016, pp 383–384.
- Gill KA: Gynecology. In Gill KA: *Ultrasound in Obstetrics and Gynecology: A Practitioner's Guide*. Pasadena, CA, Davies Publishing, 2014, pp 54–55.

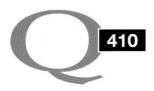

A 65-year-old postmenopausal patient presents with sudden onset of vaginal bleeding. She is not on hormone replacement therapy and has been asymptomatic for gynecologic problems. Endovaginal sonography produces the findings seen in this image. The most likely diagnosis is:

a. endometrial carcinoma
b. degenerating fibroid
c. early intrauterine pregnancy
d. adenomyosis

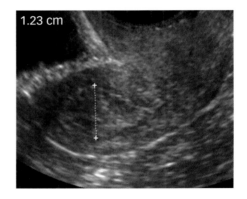

Gynecology / Postmenopausal / AIT—PACSim

A 410

A. Endometrial carcinoma.

Postmenopausal bleeding should always be evaluated when there is a suspicion of endometrial hyperplasia or endometrial cancer. After the onset of menopause and in the absence of estrogen replacement, the endometrial lining should be less than 5 mm in thickness. For a patient on hormone replacement, the thickness should not exceed 8 mm.

▶ Baun J: *Ob/Gyn Sonography: An Illustrated Review*. Pasadena, CA, Davies Publishing, 2016, pp 380–383.

Which of the following types of gynecologic malignancy is associated with the highest mortality rate?

a. cervical carcinoma
b. endometrial carcinoma
c. ovarian carcinoma
d. renal carcinoma

Gynecology / Postmenopausal

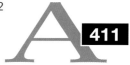

C. Ovarian carcinoma.

Ovarian carcinoma comprises about 25% of all gynecologic malignancies and is the fourth leading cause of cancer deaths in women. Its typically late diagnosis leads to its high mortality rate.

▶ Salem S: Gynecology. In Rumack CM (ed): *Diagnostic Ultrasound*, 4th edition. St. Louis, Mosby, 2011, pp 547–612.

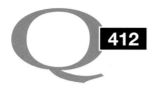

412

This patient is a 51-year-old woman with vaginal bleeding. A mass was seen on colposcopy. What is the important finding in this black-and-white version of a coronal endovaginal ultrasound using color flow?

a. ovarian mass
b. ectopic pregnancy
c. endocervical polyp
d. free fluid

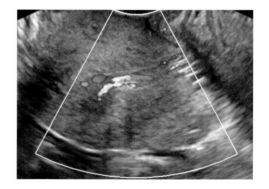

Gynecology / Postmenopausal

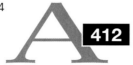

C. Endocervical polyp.

The ultrasound image presents an area within the cervical canal with color flow. The history states that a mass was seen on colposcopy, which is direct visualization of the cervix. Endocervical polyps may protrude from the cervical canal and may cause bleeding. The other choices listed do not fit with the clinical history or ultrasound image.

▶ Baun J: *Ob/Gyn Sonography: An Illustrated Review*. Pasadena, CA, Davies Publishing, 2016, pp 383–384.

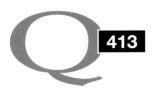

825

What term refers to a spectrum of congenital anatomic abnormalities resulting from the failed fusion of the paired embryonic paramesonephric ducts?

a. genitourinary anomalies
b. Asherman syndrome
c. Gartner's duct anomalies
d. müllerian duct anomalies

Gynecology / Pelvic Pathology

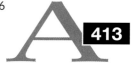

D. Müllerian duct anomalies.

The müllerian ducts are responsible for the formation of the uterus, fallopian tubes, and upper vagina. A problem with the formation of these organs may be called a *müllerian duct anomaly.*

▶ Baun J: *Ob/Gyn Sonography: An Illustrated Review*. Pasadena, CA, Davies Publishing, 2016, pp 373–375.

Total failure of fusion of the müllerian ducts results in:

a. septate uterus
b. bicornuate uterus
c. arcuate uterus
d. uterus didelphys

Gynecology / Pelvic Pathology

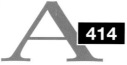

D. Uterus didelphys.

Unlike a bicornuate uterus, a *didelphic uterus* (*uterus didelphys*) comprises two distinct uteri with two cervices (*bicornuate bicollis*). In addition, there may be a vaginal septum separating the vagina into two cavities.

▶ Baun J: *Ob/Gyn Sonography: An Illustrated Review*. Pasadena, CA, Davies Publishing, 2016, pp 373–374.
▶ Hutson F: Congenital anomalies of the female genital system. In Raatz Stephenson S (ed): *Diagnostic Medical Sonography: Obstetrics and Gynecology*, 3rd edition. Philadelphia, Lippincott Williams & Wilkins, 2012, ch 3.

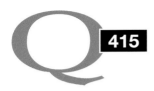

This transverse view of the uterus is diagnostic for:

a. septate uterus
b. bicornuate uterus
c. uterus didelphys
d. arcuate uterus

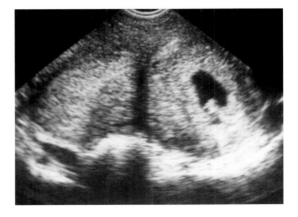

Gynecology / Pelvic Pathology

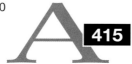

B. Bicornuate uterus.

Bicornuate uterus results from partial failure of the müllerian ducts to fuse. This results in two horns with one cervix entering into one vagina. There is a notch on the fundus of the uterus and the transverse view has a heart-shaped appearance. Two distinct endometria are noted. It may be difficult to differentiate bicornuate uterus from uterus didelphys without examining the cervix.

▶ Baun J: *Ob/Gyn Sonography: An Illustrated Review*. Pasadena, CA, Davies Publishing, 2016, pp 373–374.
▶ Hutson F: Congenital anomalies of the female genital system. In Raatz Stephenson S (ed): *Diagnostic Medical Sonography: Obstetrics and Gynecology*, 3rd edition. Philadelphia, Lippincott Williams & Wilkins, 2012, ch 3.
▶ Salem S: Gynecology. In Rumack CM (ed): *Diagnostic Ultrasound*, 4th edition. St. Louis, Mosby, 2011, pp 547–612.

831

What term is used to refer to the presence of a single uterine horn that may or may not communicate with the cervix?

a. arcuate uterus
b. bicornuate uterus
c. unicornuate uterus
d. didelphic uterus

Gynecology / Pelvic Pathology

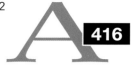

C. Unicornuate uterus.

The unicornuate uterus has one horn, similar to the mythical unicorn. In this case, there is a single, smaller uterine horn and possibly a rudimentary horn as well.

▶ Baun J: *Ob/Gyn Sonography: An Illustrated Review*. Pasadena, CA, Davies Publishing, 2016, p 373.

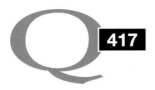

833

The round anechoic structures seen in this transvaginal image most likely represent:

a. Gartner's duct cysts
b. nabothian cysts
c. a cervical ectopic pregnancy
d. leiomyomas

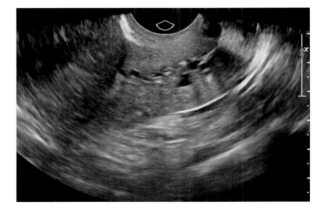

Gynecology / Pelvic Pathology

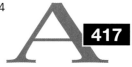

B. Nabothian cysts.

A *nabothian cyst* is a retention cyst from cervical secretions of no clinical importance and is usually asymptomatic—although a large nabothian cyst from cervical stenosis could cause pain secondary to infection.

- Baun J: *Ob/Gyn Sonography: An Illustrated Review*. Pasadena, CA, Davies Publishing, 2016, p 372.
- Gill KA: Gynecology. In Gill KA: *Ultrasound in Obstetrics and Gynecology: A Practitioner's Guide*. Pasadena, CA, Davies Publishing, pp 44–45.

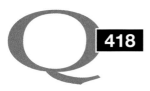

835

What is the least common type of leiomyoma but the one causing the most symptoms because of its location in relationship to the endometrium?

a. submucosal leiomyoma
b. cervical leiomyoma
c. intramural leiomyoma
d. subserosal leiomyoma

Gynecology / Pelvic Pathology

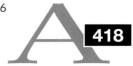

A. Submucosal leiomyoma.

Submucosal leiomyomas indent into the endometrial cavity. They are more likely to cause problems, such as bleeding and infertility, because of their relationship to the endometrium.

▶ Baun J: *Ob/Gyn Sonography: An Illustrated Review*. Pasadena, CA, Davies Publishing, 2016, pp 376–377.
▶ Gill KA: Gynecology. In Gill KA: *Ultrasound in Obstetrics and Gynecology: A Practitioner's Guide*. Pasadena, CA, Davies Publishing, 2014, pp 45–47, 50, 55–56.

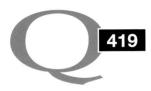

What is the echogenic structure (arrow) seen in this first trimester sonogram?

a. ectopic pregnancy
b. calcified fibroid
c. twin pregnancy demise
d. calcified arcuate arteries

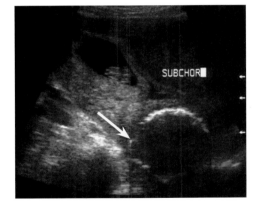

Gynecology / Pelvic Pathology

837

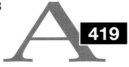

B. Calcified fibroid.

Fibroids that are calcified are degenerating. Shadowing from the calcifications may make identification of pelvic structures more difficult.

- Baun J: *Ob/Gyn Sonography: An Illustrated Review*. Pasadena, CA, Davies Publishing, 2016, pp 377–378.
- Gill KA: Gynecology. In Gill KA: *Ultrasound in Obstetrics and Gynecology: A Practitioner's Guide*. Pasadena, CA, Davies Publishing, 2014, pp 48–49.

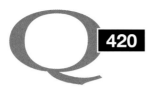 420

Masses of endometrial tissue projecting out from the surface of the endometrium and into the endometrial cavity are called:

a. endometrial carcinoma
b. endometrial polyps
c. fibroids
d. adhesions

Gynecology / Pelvic Pathology

A 420

B. Endometrial polyps.

Polyps, which may be benign or malignant, are readily seen on transvaginal ultrasound especially in the presence of endometrial fluid. Without endometrial fluid they are harder to visualize, but they may appear as a thickened endometrium.

▶ Baun J: *Ob/Gyn Sonography: An Illustrated Review*. Pasadena, CA, Davies Publishing, 2016, p 383.

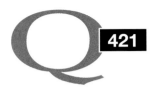

A 37-year-old woman presents with heavy menstrual periods and complains of dyspareunia. A pelvic exam reveals a symmetrically enlarged uterus with normal contours. Endovaginal sonography produces this image. The most likely diagnosis is:

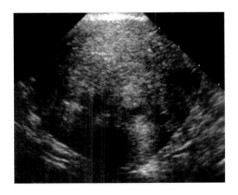

a. adenomyosis
b. endometrial carcinoma
c. choriocarcinoma
d. subserosal fibroids

Gynecology / Pelvic Pathology / AIT—PACSim

A. Adenomyosis.

Adenomyosis is endometriosis within the myometrium. With adenomyosis, the endometrium usually appears ill-defined, and there are linear shadows coming from the uterus.

▶ Baun J: *Ob/Gyn Sonography: An Illustrated Review*. Pasadena, CA, Davies Publishing, 2016, p 379.

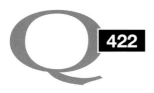

Excessive proliferation of endometrial tissue without invasion of the myometrium is called:

a. adenomyosis
b. choriocarcinoma
c. endometrial hyperplasia
d. Asherman syndrome

Gynecology / Pelvic Pathology

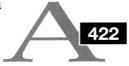

C. Endometrial hyperplasia.

Endometrial hyperplasia is thickening of the endometrium without malignancy. It is the most common cause of uterine bleeding. Sampling of the endometrium is usually indicated because it is not possible to differentiate hyperplasia from carcinoma sonographically.

▶ Baun J: *Ob/Gyn Sonography: An Illustrated Review*. Pasadena, CA, Davies Publishing, 2016, p 380.

This image demonstrates a/an:

a. cervical fibroid
b. submucosal fibroid
c. interstitial fibroid
d. subserosal fibroid

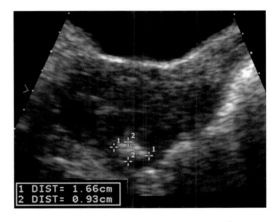

Gynecology / Pelvic Pathology

A **423**

D. Subserosal fibroid.

The calcification seen in the posterior uterus is a fibroid located just deep to the more superficial layer of the uterus, the serosal layer. A submucosal fibroid would be located within the uterine canal, and a cervical fibroid would be within the cervix.

▶ Baun J: *Ob/Gyn Sonography: An Illustrated Review*. Pasadena, CA, Davies Publishing, 2016, pp 376–377.

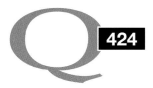

A 42-year-old patient presents with lower abdominal pain, dyspareunia, and dysmenorrhea for several months. The uterus is firm and enlarged on pelvic examination. This image is most consistent with:

a. fetus papyraceus
b. dysgerminoma
c. calcified fibroid
d. pseudomyxoma peritonei

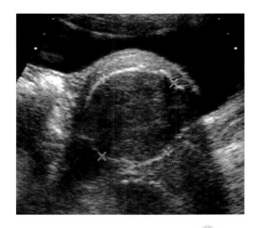

Gynecology / Pelvic Pathology / AIT—PACSim

A 424

C. Calcified fibroid.

This image is typical for a calcified fibroid. The fibroid is large and occupies most of the uterus.

▶ Baun J: *Ob/Gyn Sonography: An Illustrated Review*. Pasadena, CA, Davies Publishing, 2016, pp 377–378.

Of the following, which is the most common ovarian tumor seen in patients under 30 years of age?

a. cystadenoma
b. fibroma
c. cystic teratoma
d. dysgerminoma

Gynecology / Pelvic Pathology

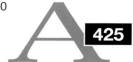

C. Cystic teratoma.

Cystic teratomas (also known as *mature* or *mature cystic* teratomas and sometimes called *dermoids*) are the most common ovarian tumor in women younger than 30, and most are benign. The *dysgerminoma* is a solid malignant tumor seen in the 20- to 30-year-old age group and is rare. The other tumors are seen primarily in peri- and postmenopausal women.

- Baun J: *Ob/Gyn Sonography: An Illustrated Review*. Pasadena, CA, Davies Publishing, 2016, p 392.
- Gill KA: Gynecology. In Gill KA: *Ultrasound in Obstetrics and Gynecology: A Practitioner's Guide*. Pasadena, CA, Davies Publishing, 2014, pp 67–69.

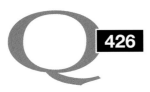

MOST ovarian tumors are:

a. solid
b. benign
c. malignant
d. androgenic

Gynecology / Pelvic Pathology

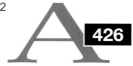

B. Benign.

Of all ovarian neoplasms, 80% are benign. The most common ovarian neoplasm in women under the age of 30 is the dermoid, or mature cystic teratoma. The most common neoplasm in reproductive and menopausal women is the cystadenoma, which is predominantly cystic and also benign. Solid, malignant, and androgenic tumors, in general, are not common.

- Baun J: *Ob/Gyn Sonography: An Illustrated Review*. Pasadena, CA, Davies Publishing, 2016, p 384.
- Gill KA: Gynecology. In Gill KA: *Ultrasound in Obstetrics and Gynecology: A Practitioner's Guide*. Pasadena, CA, Davies Publishing, 2014, p 66.
- Raatz Stephenson S (ed): *Diagnostic Medical Sonography: Obstetrics and Gynecology*, 3rd edition. Baltimore, Lippincott Williams & Wilkins, 2012, p 198.

853

A patient presenting with a history of amenorrhea, hirsutism, obesity, hypertension, and infertility is at risk for:

a. polycystic ovaries
b. paraovarian cysts
c. theca-lutein cysts
d. ovarian hyperstimulation syndrome

Gynecology / Pelvic Pathology

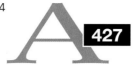

A. Polycystic ovaries.

A patient with classic *polycystic ovary syndrome* (also known as *Stein-Leventhal syndrome*) presents with hirsutism, obesity, and amenorrhea. The patient may also have infertility.

- Baun J: *Ob/Gyn Sonography: An Illustrated Review*. Pasadena, CA, Davies Publishing, 2016, p 388.
- Gill KA: Gynecology. In Gill KA: *Ultrasound in Obstetrics and Gynecology: A Practitioner's Guide*. Pasadena, CA, Davies Publishing, 2014, p 59.

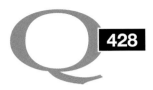

855

The sonographic findings in this image are most consistent with:

a. Sertoli-Leydig tumor
b. cystadenocarcinoma
c. dysgerminoma
d. mature cystic teratoma

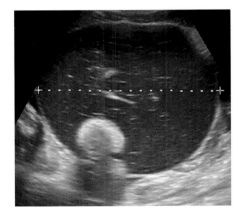

Gynecology / Pelvic Pathology

A 428

D. Mature cystic teratoma.

The *mature cystic teratoma*, or *dermoid*, has a widely variable appearance. A common appearance is that of a cystic mass with solid components. These masses are usually benign and may contain hair, teeth, and solid tissues. *Dysgerminomas* and *Sertoli-Leydig tumors* are usually solid. *Cystadenocarcinomas* may have septations but otherwise are usually cystic. See also the answer to question 425.

▶ Baun J: *Ob/Gyn Sonography: An Illustrated Review*. Pasadena, CA, Davies Publishing, 2016, p 392.

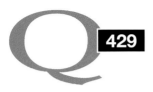

Q 429

The functional, non-neoplastic enlargement of an ovary caused by failure of the dominant follicle to regress after ovulation is called a:

a. theca-lutein cyst
b. follicular cyst
c. hemorrhagic cyst
d. corpus luteum cyst

Gynecology / Pelvic Pathology

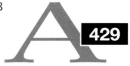

D. Corpus luteum cyst.

If the corpus luteum does not involute after ovulation, a corpus luteum cyst is formed. These cysts, compared to follicular cysts, tend to be thick-walled and sometimes hemorrhagic. When interrogated using Doppler color flow imaging, corpus luteum cysts may appear with a rim of color flow around them.

- Baun J: *Ob/Gyn Sonography: An Illustrated Review*. Pasadena, CA, Davies Publishing, 2016, p 385.
- Hagen-Ansert SL (ed): *Textbook of Diagnostic Ultrasonography*, 7th edition. St. Louis, Elsevier Mosby, 2012, p 1007.

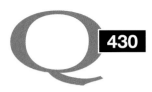

Q 430

The most common histologic type of malignant ovarian neoplasm is:

a. Brenner tumor
b. thecoma
c. dysgerminoma
d. cystadenocarcinoma

Gynecology / Pelvic Pathology

A **430**

D. Cystadenocarcinoma.

Cystadenocarcinoma is the most common type of ovarian cancer. Ovarian cancer is called a "silent killer" because these tumors can grow very large before they are identified, and by the time they are diagnosed they frequently have already metastasized.

▶ Baun J: *Ob/Gyn Sonography: An Illustrated Review*. Pasadena, CA, Davies Publishing, 2016, pp 390–391.
▶ Gill KA: Gynecology. In Gill KA: *Ultrasound in Obstetrics and Gynecology: A Practitioner's Guide*. Pasadena, CA, Davies Publishing, 2014, p 71.

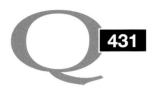

861

A 50-year-old woman presents complaining of generalized malaise and a full feeling in her abdomen. Her CA-125 serum assay is elevated. Given this history, this image is most consistent with:

a. ovarian cystadenocarcinoma
b. hemorrhagic ovarian cyst
c. dysgerminoma
d. pelvic inflammatory disease

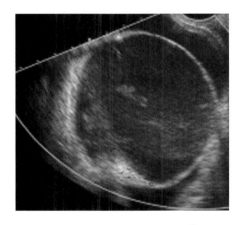

Gynecology / Pelvic Pathology / AIT—PACSim

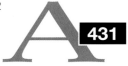

A. Ovarian cystadenocarcinoma.

Given the clinical history and image provided, the most likely diagnosis is ovarian cancer. Serous cystadenocarcinoma is the most common type of ovarian cancer.

▶ Baun J: *Ob/Gyn Sonography: An Illustrated Review*. Pasadena, CA, Davies Publishing, 2016, pp 390–391.

This is an image of the abdomen of a 52-year-old woman with a large ovarian mass. The image has a sonographic feature that is consistent with what pathology?

a. ovarian cancer
b. ruptured ectopic pregnancy
c. pelvic inflammatory disease
d. adnexal cyst

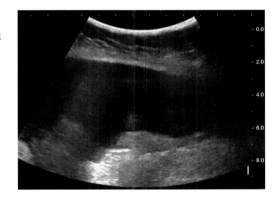

Gynecology / Pelvic Pathology / AIT—PACSim

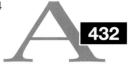

A. Ovarian cancer.

This image presents a finding called an "omental cake," which appears as thickening of the anterior abdominal wall with ascites and is commonly associated with peritoneal seeding from ovarian cancer.

- Baun J: *Ob/Gyn Sonography: An Illustrated Review*. Pasadena, CA, Davies Publishing, 2016, pp 388–397.
- Raatz Stephenson S (ed): *Diagnostic Medical Sonography: Obstetrics and Gynecology*, 3rd edition. Baltimore, Lippincott Williams & Wilkins, 2012, ch 10.

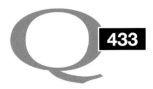

A 26-year-old female with a negative beta-hCG titer was sent in for left-lower-quadrant pain. The structure imaged below was found in the patient's right lower quadrant. What is the most likely diagnosis?

a. tubo-ovarian abscess
b. ovarian cancer
c. benign cystic teratoma
d. ectopic pregnancy

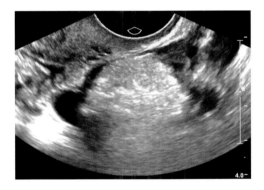

Gynecology / Pelvic Pathology / AIT—PACSim

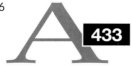

C. Benign cystic teratoma.

The *mature cystic teratoma*, often called a *dermoid tumor* or *dermoid cyst*, is a benign mass made up of all three germ layers. It usually does not cause pain, although it may torse the ovary and cause pain through torsion. On ultrasound a dermoid looks like a complex echogenic mass with shadowing due to the hair and other materials that may be found in the dermoid.

▶ Baun J: *Ob/Gyn Sonography: An Illustrated Review*. Pasadena, CA, Davies Publishing, 2016, pp 392–393.
▶ Gill KA: Gynecology. In Gill KA: *Ultrasound in Obstetrics and Gynecology: A Practitioner's Guide*. Pasadena, CA, Davies Publishing, 2014, p 67.

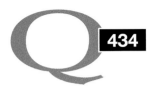

A 38-year-old patient with a history of endometriosis presents with dysuria, dyspareunia, low back pain, and heavy periods. This image most likely represents:

a. hemorrhagic corpus luteum cyst
b. Brenner tumor
c. endometrial carcinoma
d. endometrioma

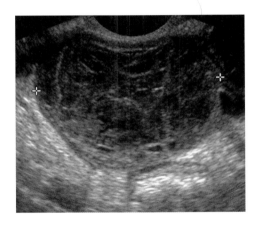

Gynecology / Pelvic Pathology / AIT—PACSim

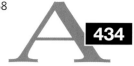

D. Endometrioma.

Endometriomas—sometimes referred to as "chocolate cysts"—are complex masses of the adnexa resulting from ectopic endometrial implants, known as *endometriosis*. Hemorrhagic cysts can have a similar appearance, but the clinical history makes endometrioma most likely.

▶ Baun J: *Ob/Gyn Sonography: An Illustrated Review*. Pasadena, CA, Davies Publishing, 2016, p 399–400.

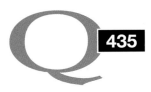

Which of the following may cause endometriosis?

a. infertility
b. retrograde menses
c. obesity
d. decreased levels of estrogen

Gynecology / Pelvic Pathology

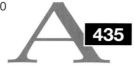

B. Retrograde menses.

Although theories abound regarding the cause of endometriosis, one theory involves spillage of the menses via the fallopian tubes into the adnexa. Infertility may result from endometriosis.

- Baun J: *Ob/Gyn Sonography: An Illustrated Review*. Pasadena, CA, Davies Publishing, 2016, p 399.
- Cowett AA: Pelvic inflammatory disease and endometriosis. In Raatz Stephenson S (ed): *Diagnostic Medical Sonography: Obstetrics and Gynecology*, 3rd edition. Philadelphia, Lippincott Williams & Wilkins, 2012, ch 11.

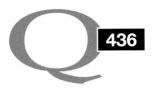

Q 436

An obese patient presents with a history of infertility and hirsutism. Sonography produces this image. The most likely diagnosis is:

a. polycystic ovaries
b. ovarian torsion
c. theca-lutein cysts
d. anovulatory cysts

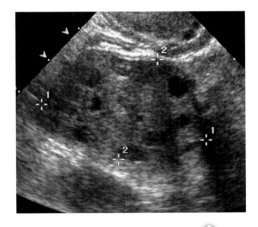

Gynecology / Pelvic Pathology / AIT—PACSim

A 436

A. Polycystic ovaries.

The clinical picture is suggestive of polycystic ovary syndrome (PCOS). The image shows a rounded ovary with peripherally located follicles, also suggestive of PCOS.

▶ Baun J: *Ob/Gyn Sonography: An Illustrated Review*. Pasadena, CA, Davies Publishing, 2016, p 388.

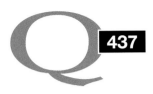

An enlarged ovary with a rounded shape and peripherally located follicles in a "string of pearls" configuration is suggestive of what condition?

a. theca-lutein cysts
b. hemorrhagic cysts
c. ovarian hyperstimulation syndrome
d. Stein-Leventhal syndrome

Gynecology / Pelvic Pathology

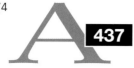

D. Stein-Leventhal syndrome.

Stein-Leventhal syndrome is also called *polycystic ovary syndrome* (PCOS). It is characterized clinically by excess facial hair (hirsutism), infertility, obesity, and anovulation. None of the other choices listed presents as a "string of pearls."

▶ Baun J: *Ob/Gyn Sonography: An Illustrated Review*. Pasadena, CA, Davies Publishing, 2016, pp 388, 411.
▶ Gill KA: Gynecology. In Gill KA: *Ultrasound in Obstetrics and Gynecology: A Practitioner's Guide*. Pasadena, CA, Davies Publishing, 2014, pp 59–60.

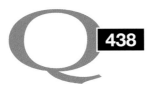

The condition in which the fallopian tube is distended with pus is called:

a. pyosalpinx
b. hydrosalpinx
c. tubo-ovarian abscess
d. salpingitis

Gynecology / Pelvic Pathology

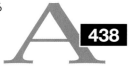

A. Pyosalpinx.

The root *pyo* means pus. A *tubo-ovarian abscess* (TOA) may or may not be present with a pyosalpinx. *Salpingitis* is inflammation of the tube, and *hydrosalpinx* is fluid within the tube.

- Baun J: *Ob/Gyn Sonography: An Illustrated Review*. Pasadena, CA, Davies Publishing, 2016, p 398.
- Cowett AA: Pelvic inflammatory disease and endometriosis. In Raatz Stephenson S (ed): *Diagnostic Medical Sonography: Obstetrics and Gynecology*, 3rd edition. Philadelphia, Lippincott Williams & Wilkins, 2012, ch 11.

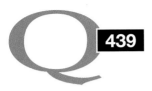

439

In pelvic inflammatory disease, an inflammatory mass extending beyond the fallopian tubes is called:

a. pyosalpinx
b. hydrosalpinx
c. tubal carcinoma
d. tubo-ovarian abscess

Gynecology / Pelvic Pathology

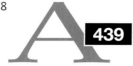

D. Tubo-ovarian abscess.

These patients will present with fever, shaking chills, acute pain, increased white blood cell count, and Fitz-Hugh–Curtis syndrome. A tubo-ovarian abscess (TOA) is classified as stage III pelvic inflammatory disease (PID).

▶ Baun J: *Ob/Gyn Sonography: An Illustrated Review*. Pasadena, CA, Davies Publishing, 2016, pp 398–399.
▶ Cowett AA: Pelvic inflammatory disease and endometriosis. In Raatz Stephenson S (ed): *Diagnostic Medical Sonography: Obstetrics and Gynecology*, 3rd edition. Philadelphia, Lippincott Williams & Wilkins, 2012, ch 11.

A patient presents with a normal last menstrual period 2 weeks ago, a fever, leukocytosis, and a fluid collection in the cul-de-sac. The most likely diagnosis is:

a. tubo-ovarian abscess
b. ruptured ectopic pregnancy
c. ascites
d. follicular cyst

Gynecology / Pelvic Pathology

A 440

A. Tubo-ovarian abscess.

For a diagnosis of tubo-ovarian abscess (TOA), there should be a history of pelvic inflammatory disease (PID) or clinical symptoms consistent with infection. Clinical symptoms would include fever, pain, and increased white blood cell count (leukocytosis). The clinical history of fever and leukocytosis is the key factor.

▶ Baun J: *Ob/Gyn Sonography: An Illustrated Review*. Pasadena, CA, Davies Publishing, 2016, pp 398–399.

▶ Gill KA: Gynecology. In Gill KA: *Ultrasound in Obstetrics and Gynecology: A Practitioner's Guide*. Pasadena, CA, Davies Publishing, 2014, pp 63–64.

Acute inflammation of the uterine lining is called:

a. endometritis
b. parametritis
c. pelvic inflammatory disease
d. peritonitis

Gynecology / Pelvic Pathology

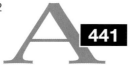

A. Endometritis.

Endometritis is inflammation of the uterine lining. Infection may spread from the endometrium to the tubes. Endometritis is a stage of pelvic inflammatory disease.

▶ Baun J: *Ob/Gyn Sonography: An Illustrated Review*. Pasadena, CA, Davies Publishing, 2016, p 381.

A 29-year-old patient presents with fever and an elevated white blood cell count and complains of severe pain in her left lower quadrant. This image is most consistent with a diagnosis of:

a. ruptured ovarian cyst
b. ovarian torsion
c. ectopic pregnancy
d. pelvic inflammatory disease

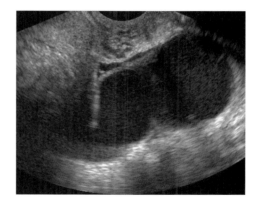

Gynecology / Pelvic Pathology / AIT—PACSim

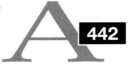

D. Pelvic inflammatory disease.

Although this image is nonspecific and could represent an adnexal mass, ovarian cyst, or hydrosalpinx, the clinical history (fever and leukocytosis) suggests infection or pelvic inflammatory disease (PID).

▶ Baun J: *Ob/Gyn Sonography: An Illustrated Review*. Pasadena, CA, Davies Publishing, 2016, pp 398–399.

Doppler flow within a suspected ovarian malignancy becomes a concern when:

a. The resistivity index is less than 0.4.
b. The resistivity index is greater than 0.4.
c. The pulsatility index is greater than 1.
d. The pulsatility index is less than 0.5.

Gynecology / Pelvic Pathology

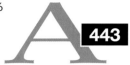

A. The resistivity index is less than 0.4.

Doppler findings are concerning when the resistivity index is less than 0.4 and the pulsatility index is less than 1.0. Although the indices do not define benign or malignant, they may be used in conjunction with the clinical history and sonographic findings.

▶ Raatz Stephenson S (ed): *Diagnostic Medical Sonography: Obstetrics and Gynecology*, 3rd edition. Baltimore, Lippincott Williams & Wilkins, 2012, ch 6.

In the evaluation of pelvic pathology, color Doppler may be used to evaluate:

a. peak systolic and end-diastolic velocities
b. presence of flow
c. resistivity indices
d. pulsatility indices

Gynecology / Pelvic Pathology

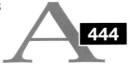

B. Presence of flow.

Color Doppler obtains only mean velocity information and therefore is unable to provide information on peak systolic or end-diastolic velocities. It can, however, establish presence of flow and provide information about direction of flow.

- Baun J: *Ob/Gyn Sonography: An Illustrated Review*. Pasadena, CA, Davies Publishing, 2016, p 447.
- Baun J: Doppler applications in obstetric and gynecologic sonography. In Gill KA: *Ultrasound in Obstetrics and Gynecology: A Practitioner's Guide*. Pasadena, CA, Davies Publishing, 2014, p 374.

Which of the following is the invasive x-ray test used to visualize the uterus and fallopian tubes?

a. intravenous pyelogram
b. hysterosalpingogram
c. angiogram
d. myelogram

Gynecology / Pelvic Pathology

A 445

B. Hysterosalpingogram.

Hysterosalpingography (HSG) is a test that uses ionizing radiation and a radiopaque dye instilled into the uterus through the cervix in order to opacify the endometrial canal and fallopian tubes. Before ultrasound it was the only imaging exam to rule out polyps in the endometrium and check tubal patency.

▶ Baun J: *Ob/Gyn Sonography: An Illustrated Review*. Pasadena, CA, Davies Publishing, 2016, p 472.

▶ Bega G: Volume sonography. In Gill KA: *Ultrasound in Obstetrics and Gynecology: A Practitioner's Guide*. Pasadena, CA, Davies Publishing, 2014, p 430.

891

446

What is the office-based procedure that may be performed by a gynecologist to visualize the cervix in more detail?

a. vulvoplasty
b. pyelogram
c. colposcopy
d. hysterogram

Gynecology / Pelvic Pathology

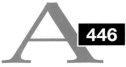

C. Colposcopy.

Colposcopy is a procedure performed in the gynecologist's office that permits direct visualization of the cervix. A tissue sample for cervical biopsy is usually collected at this point.

▶ Raatz Stephenson S (ed): *Diagnostic Medical Sonography: Obstetrics and Gynecology*, 3rd edition. Baltimore, Lippincott Williams & Wilkins, 2012, ch 9.

893

How should the endometrium be measured in the presence of endometrial fluid?

a. The entire thickness should be measured, including the hypoechoic border.
b. From anterior basal layer to posterior basal layer, including the fluid.
c. From anterior basal layer to the fluid, and from posterior basal layer to the fluid.
d. Only the fluid is measured.

Gynecology / Pelvic Pathology

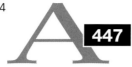

C. From anterior basal layer to the fluid, and from posterior basal layer to the fluid.

The endometrium should be measured from the echogenic basal layer to the fluid anteriorly and posteriorly. The hypoechoic area next to the basal layer should be part of the measurement. Do not include endometrial fluid in the measurement.

- Baun J: *Ob/Gyn Sonography: An Illustrated Review*. Pasadena, CA, Davies Publishing, 2016, p 500.
- Gill KA: Gynecology. In Gill KA: *Ultrasound in Obstetrics and Gynecology: A Practitioner's Guide*. Pasadena, CA, Davies Publishing, 2014, pp 34–35, p 519.

What is the reason the endometrium is being measured as displayed in this image?

a. This endometrium has been measured incorrectly.
b. There is an IUD present.
c. There is an intrauterine mass.
d. There is endometrial fluid.

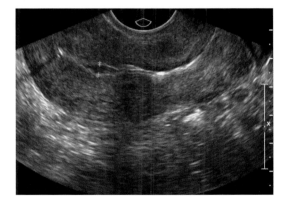

Gynecology / Pelvic Pathology

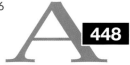

D. There is endometrial fluid.

In the presence of endometrial fluid, the endometrium has to be measured in a way that does not include the fluid in the measurement, as seen in this image.

- Baun J: *Ob/Gyn Sonography: An Illustrated Review*. Pasadena, CA, Davies Publishing, 2016, p 500.
- Gill KA: Ultrasound in *Obstetrics and Gynecology: A Practitioner's Guide*. Pasadena, CA, Davies Publishing, 2014, pp 52, 519.

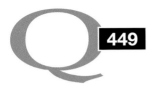

This patient has a negative serum beta-hCG and severe left-lower-quadrant pain. What is the most likely diagnosis?

a. ectopic pregnancy
b. ruptured hemorrhagic ovarian cyst
c. intrauterine pregnancy
d. dermoid tumor

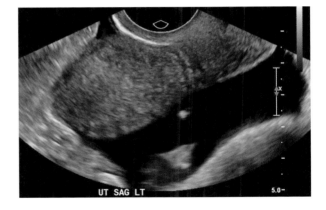

Gynecology / Pelvic Pathology

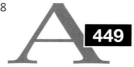

B. Ruptured hemorrhagic ovarian cyst.

With a negative serum beta-hCG, this patient cannot have a pregnancy inside or outside of the uterus. Given the moderate amount of cul-de-sac fluid, a ruptured hemorrhagic cyst should be suspected. A patient with a ruptured hemorrhagic ovarian cyst can decompensate as much as a patient with a ruptured ectopic pregnancy if there is active bleeding. Free fluid is not an indication of a dermoid.

▶ Baun J: *Ob/Gyn Sonography: An Illustrated Review*. Pasadena, CA, Davies Publishing, 2016, pp 386–387.
▶ Gill KA: Gynecology. In Gill KA: *Ultrasound in Obstetrics and Gynecology: A Practitioner's Guide*. Pasadena, CA, Davies Publishing, 2014, pp 57–58.

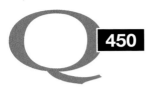

450

The condition associated with ascites and a right pleural effusion in a patient with a solid benign tumor is:

a. Stein-Leventhal syndrome
b. Meigs syndrome
c. Beckwith-Wiedemann syndrome
d. Edwards syndrome

Gynecology / Extrapelvic Pathology

A 450

B. Meigs syndrome.

Meigs syndrome is usually caused by a fibroma and is associated with right pleural effusion and ascites.

▶ Gill KA: Gynecology. In Gill KA: *Ultrasound in Obstetrics and Gynecology: A Practitioner's Guide*. Pasadena, CA, Davies Publishing, 2014, p 70.

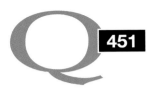

451

A patient presents with shoulder pain, a positive beta-hCG titer, an empty uterus, and free fluid in the cul-de-sac demonstrated with ultrasound. You should also scan:

a. the kidneys to rule out hydronephrosis
b. the right upper quadrant to rule out fluid in Morison's pouch
c. the gallbladder to rule out stones
d. the heart to rule out pericardial effusion

Gynecology / Extrapelvic Pathology / AIT—PACSim

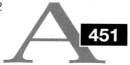

A 451

B. The right upper quadrant to rule out fluid in Morison's pouch.

An ectopic pregnancy that has ruptured will lead to blood spreading first in the posterior cul-de-sac because of its dependent position. Excessive blood will spread retrograde and follow specific pathways. The space between the right kidney and the liver is a common space for fluid collections.

▶ Gill KA: *Ultrasound in Obstetrics and Gynecology: A Practitioner's Guide*. Pasadena, CA, Davies Publishing, 2014, pp 73, 109, 467.

903

Your patient has a history of treatment for ovarian cancer. Which blood test is used to determine her status?

a. CA-125
b. beta-hCG
c. FSH
d. TSH

Gynecology / Extrapelvic Pathology

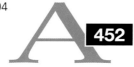

A. CA-125.

The CA-125 test is used to test for a recurrence of ovarian cancer in a patient previously treated for ovarian cancer. Rising levels in serial CA-125 tests may indicate a recurrence.

- Baun J: *Ob/Gyn Sonography: An Illustrated Review*. Pasadena, CA, Davies Publishing, 2016, pp 390, 431–432.
- Gill KA: Gynecology. In Gill KA: *Ultrasound in Obstetrics and Gynecology: A Practitioner's Guide*. Pasadena, CA, Davies Publishing, 2014, p 72.

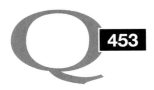

453

A patient presents with abdominal swelling, low back pain, and an extremely elevated CA-125. Evaluation of her right upper quadrant indicates:

a. normal liver
b. metastatic liver disease
c. perihepatitis
d. liver abscess

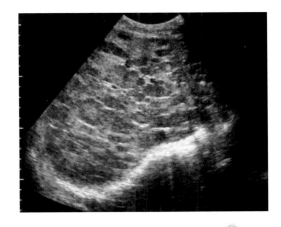

Gynecology / Extrapelvic Pathology / AIT—PACSim

A

453

B. Metastatic liver disease.

Ovarian malignancies can metastasize to distant sites, including the liver as seen here. Other characteristics that raise suspicion for a malignant pelvic mass include ascites, an irregular anterior abdominal wall with a solid component, and pelvic lymphadenopathy.

▶ Baun J: *Ob/Gyn Sonography: An Illustrated Review*. Pasadena, CA, Davies Publishing, 2016, pp 390, 431–432, 471.

▶ Gill KA: Gynecology. In Gill KA: *Ultrasound in Obstetrics and Gynecology: A Practitioner's Guide*. Pasadena, CA, Davies Publishing, 2014, pp 71–73.

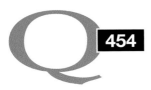

Ultrasound demonstrates the presence of a large leiomyoma in your patient. You should also scan the:

a. liver
b. kidneys
c. peritoneal cavity
d. aorta

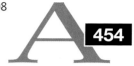

B. Kidneys.

Large leiomyomas can cause compression of the ureters, leading to hydronephrosis of the kidneys. Both kidneys should be evaluated if a large leiomyoma is visualized.

▶ Raatz Stephenson S (ed): *Diagnostic Medical Sonography: Obstetrics and Gynecology*, 3rd edition. Baltimore, Lippincott Williams & Wilkins, 2012, ch 8.

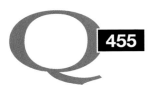

455

What pathology may result from large pelvic masses compressing a ureter?

a. liver congestion
b. uterine prolapse
c. hydronephrosis
d. vaginal atrophy

Gynecology / Extrapelvic Pathology

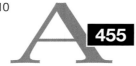

C. Hydronephrosis.

Hydronephrosis is a backup of fluid in one or both kidneys. One cause of hydronephrosis is a pelvic mass impinging on a ureter.

- Baun J: *Ob/Gyn Sonography: An Illustrated Review*. Pasadena, CA, Davies Publishing, 2016, p 258.
- Raatz Stephenson S (ed): *Diagnostic Medical Sonography: Obstetrics and Gynecology*, 3rd edition. Baltimore, Lippincott Williams & Wilkins, 2012, ch 8.

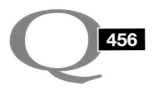

456

A 24-year-old patient presents with right-lower-quadrant pain, nausea and vomiting, and an elevated white blood cell count. The uterus and ovaries appear normal. What other etiology may account for the pain?

a. liver congestion
b. aortic aneurysm
c. hydronephrosis
d. appendicitis

Gynecology / Extrapelvic Pathology

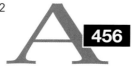

D. Appendicitis.

Appendicitis may present as right-lower-quadrant pain, an elevated white blood cell count, and nausea and vomiting. In the absence of pelvic pathology in a patient with right-lower-quadrant pain, appendicitis should be considered if the patient still has an appendix.

▶ Baun J: *Ob/Gyn Sonography: An Illustrated Review*. Pasadena, CA, Davies Publishing, 2016, p 400.
▶ Gill KA: Gynecology. In Gill KA: *Ultrasound in Obstetrics and Gynecology: A Practitioner's Guide*. Pasadena, CA, Davies Publishing, 2014, pp 65, 382.

457

Perihepatitis can be associated with pelvic inflammatory disease, causing right-upper-quadrant tenderness and pain. This condition is known as:

a. Turner syndrome
b. Stein-Leventhal syndrome
c. Meigs syndrome
d. Fitz-Hugh–Curtis syndrome

Gynecology / Extrapelvic Pathology

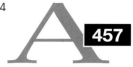

D. Fitz-Hugh–Curtis syndrome.

Near the level of the fallopian tubes there is a communication between the abdominal and pelvic compartments through which ascites and blood can migrate into the upper abdominal quadrants. If untreated, pelvic inflammation can migrate and cause inflammation around the liver, eventually leading to perihepatitis and peritonitis.

- Baun J: *Ob/Gyn Sonography: An Illustrated Review*. Pasadena, CA, Davies Publishing, 2016, p 398.
- Gill KA: Gynecology. In Gill KA: *Ultrasound in Obstetrics and Gynecology: A Practitioner's Guide*. Pasadena, CA, Davies Publishing, 2014, p 63.

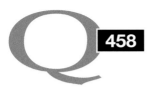

915

When trying to differentiate between an infectious process and a noninfectious process, which lab value should you examine?

a. white blood cell count
b. red blood cell count
c. amylase
d. CA-125

Patient Care, Scanning Technique, and Physical Principles

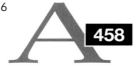

A. White blood cell count.

The white blood cell (WBC) count, when elevated, is an indicator of infection. The other values are not specific to infection.

▶ Raatz Stephenson S (ed): *Diagnostic Medical Sonography: Obstetrics and Gynecology*, 3rd edition. Baltimore, Wolters Kluwer/Lippincott Williams & Wilkins, 2012, ch 8.

917

Which of the following will give the sonographer important information related to the expected size of the patient's nonpregnant, premenopausal uterus?

a. last menstrual period
b. gravidity/parity
c. lab values
d. vaginal inspection

Patient Care, Scanning Technique, and Physical Principles

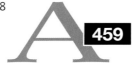

B. Gravidity/parity.

Gravidity is the condition of being pregnant (regardless of outcome); *parity* refers to a woman's condition with regard to having delivered viable offspring. The uterus varies in size depending on how many pregnancies a patient has had. A normal *nulliparous* uterus (i.e., the uterus of a woman who has not given birth) is usually smaller than a *multiparous* uterus (i.e., that of a woman who has given birth in two or more pregnancies).

▶ Raatz Stephenson S (ed): *Diagnostic Medical Sonography: Obstetrics and Gynecology*, 3rd edition. Baltimore, Lippincott Williams & Wilkins, 2012, ch 1.

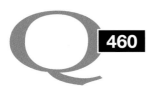

460

Your currently nonpregnant patient has been designated as G3P2102. She has given birth to how many preterm babies?

a. 0
b. 2
c. 1
d. 3

Patient Care, Scanning Technique, and Physical Principles

A 460

C. 1.

The gravidity/parity or gravida/para (GP) system works this way: G = the number of pregnancies, and P = parities by type, whether full-term, preterm, abortion, or live births. (One trick for remembering parities by type is to use the abbreviation FPAL and remember it as "Florida Power And Light.") Therefore G3P2102 would indicate three pregnancies in total, with two full-term, one preterm, none abortive, and two live births.

▶ Raatz Stephenson S (ed): *Diagnostic Medical Sonography: Obstetrics and Gynecology*, 3rd edition. Baltimore, Lippincott Williams & Wilkins, 2012, ch 1.

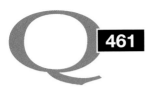

461

When reporting the results of a sonographic examination to a referring practitioner, your most important consideration is:

a. providing the information in an accurate and timely manner
b. making it clear that it is only a preliminary report
c. categorizing the report as "technical findings only"
d. obtaining interpreting physician approval first

Patient Care, Scanning Technique, and Physical Principles

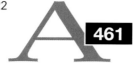

A. Providing the information in an accurate and timely manner.

When providing a report to the referring practitioner, the sonographer is relaying the final diagnosis as provided by the interpreting physician. The most important thing for the sonographer to do is to provide an accurate report in a timely fashion so that the communication of any information of an emergent nature is not delayed.

▶ Baun J: *Ob/Gyn Sonography: An Illustrated Review*. Pasadena, CA, Davies Publishing, 2016, p 471.

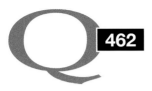

462

What is the best way to ensure patient cooperation?

a. Use a transducer of the proper frequency.
b. Perform the exam as quickly as possible.
c. Have a chaperone observe the exam.
d. Explain the exam to the patient.

Patient Care, Scanning Technique, and Physical Principles

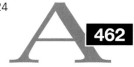

D. Explain the exam to the patient.

A patient who understands what is about to take place will be more cooperative than a patient who is confused or anxious.

- Baun J: *Ob/Gyn Sonography: An Illustrated Review*. Pasadena, CA, Davies Publishing, 2016, pp 462–463.
- Raatz Stephenson S (ed): *Diagnostic Medical Sonography: Obstetrics and Gynecology*, 3rd edition. Baltimore, Lippincott Williams & Wilkins, 2012, ch 1.

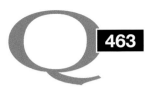

Thorough explanation of the exam to the patient may result in what beneficial side effect?

a. decreased patient complaints
b. longer exam times
c. more detailed preliminary reports
d. less costly examinations

Patient Care, Scanning Technique, and Physical Principles

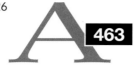

A. Decreased patient complaints.

A patient who understands what is about to happen and who is kept informed is less likely to complain than an uninformed patient. Although it may add a few minutes to the exam, explaining the procedure is better patient care.

▶ Raatz Stephenson S (ed): *Diagnostic Medical Sonography: Obstetrics and Gynecology*, 3rd edition. Baltimore, Lippincott Williams & Wilkins, 2012, ch 1.

464

Which of the following would be the best question to ask a patient in order to date the last menstrual period?

a. What is your LMP?
b. Do you know when your last menstrual period was?
c. When was the last day of your last menstrual period?
d. When was the first day of your last menstrual period?

Patient Care, Scanning Technique, and Physical Principles

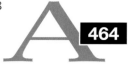

D. When was the first day of your last menstrual period?

Medical practitioners sometimes forget that patients do not know medical terminology. Most patients do not know that *last menstrual period* or LMP refers to the *first* day of the LMP and may assume it means the *end* of the last menstrual period. By asking the patient, "When was the *first day* of your last menstrual period?" you are more likely to get the information you need.

▶ Baun J: *Ob/Gyn Sonography: An Illustrated Review*. Pasadena, CA, Davies Publishing, 2016, p 69.

Your third trimester patient feels faint and nauseated during a sonographic examination. What should you do?

a. Have her lie flat and breathe deeply.
b. Have her sit up and sip water.
c. Roll her onto her left side, right side up.
d. Roll her onto her right side, left side up.

Patient Care, Scanning Technique, and Physical Principles

A 465

C. Roll her onto her left side, right side up.

Supine hypotensive syndrome is caused by excessive pressure on the inferior vena cava, which leads to a decrease in blood pressure and thus a feeling of faintness and nausea. These symptoms are usually relieved by rolling the patient onto her left side, right side up, known as the *left lateral decubitus position*.

▶ Baun J: *Ob/Gyn Sonography: An Illustrated Review*. Pasadena, CA, Davies Publishing, 2016, p 465.

▶ Gill KA: Maternal disorders and pregnancy. In Gill KA: *Ultrasound in Obstetrics and Gynecology: A Practitioner's Guide*. Pasadena, CA, Davies Publishing, 2014, p 313.

931

A method of quantifying the potential for the ultrasonic heating of human tissue is known as:

a. acoustic output
b. mechanical index
c. spatial resolution
d. thermal index

Patient Care, Scanning Technique, and Physical Principles

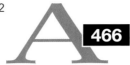

D. Thermal index.

The *thermal index* (TI) is a measure of the potential for thermal bioeffects, or heating of tissue. Fetal tissue is more sensitive to thermal bioeffects compared to adult tissue. The thermal index is calculated using the following equation:

$$TI = \frac{W_O}{W_{deg}}$$

where W_O = output power of the transducer (watts), W_{deg} = the power necessary to raise tissue temperature, and TI = a calculated estimate of temperature increase. Decreasing the acoustic output will decrease the thermal index.

▶ Baun J: *Ob/Gyn Sonography: An Illustrated Review*. Pasadena, CA, Davies Publishing, 2016, p 440.
▶ Merritt CRB: Physics of ultrasound. In Rumack CM (ed): *Diagnostic Ultrasound*, 4th edition. St. Louis, Mosby, 2011, pp 2–33.

A potential bioeffect from exposure to ultrasound waves is:

a. hematoma from transducer pressure
b. leukemia
c. tissue heating
d. There is none.

Patient Care, Scanning Technique, and Physical Principles

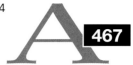

C. Tissue heating.

Human tissue absorbs the ultrasound energy. Absorption is the conversion of sound energy to heat. This bioeffect is measured using a method known as the *thermal index*.

- Baun J: *Ob/Gyn Sonography: An Illustrated Review*. Pasadena, CA, Davies Publishing, 2016, p 440.
- Kremkau FW: *Sonography: Principles and Instruments*, 9th edition. St. Louis, Elsevier, 2016, pp 221, 233–236.
- Merritt CRB: Physics of ultrasound. In Rumack CM (ed): *Diagnostic Ultrasound*, 4th edition. St. Louis, Mosby, 2011, pp 2–33.

The acronym for safe usage practices in diagnostic ultrasound is:

a. SPTA
b. SPPA
c. ALARA
d. SATA

Patient Care, Scanning Technique, and Physical Principles

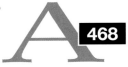

C. ALARA.

ALARA stands for "as low as reasonably achievable," which is the principle of minimizing potential risk to the patient when applying acoustic energy to the body. Practice safe diagnostic ultrasound by scanning only when indicated, keeping the output power low, not leaving the transducer over the same area longer than necessary, and reducing exposure time.

- American Institute of Ultrasound in Medicine: AIUM practice guideline for the performance of obstetric ultrasound examinations. Available at www.aium.org.
- Baun J: *Ob/Gyn Sonography: An Illustrated Review*. Pasadena, CA, Davies Publishing, 2016, p 473.
- Kremkau FW: *Sonography: Principles and Instruments*, 9th edition. St. Louis, Elsevier, 2016, pp 221, 235.

937

The mechanical index (MI) measures:

a. thermal changes in soft tissue
b. positive acoustic pressure present in a medium
c. cavitational changes
d. negative acoustic pressure present in a medium

Patient Care, Scanning Technique, and Physical Principles

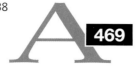

D. Negative acoustic pressure present in a medium.

The *mechanical index* (MI) is a measure of the risk for cavitational (mechanical) bioeffects. The MI is based on the *peak rarefactional pressure*, also known as the *peak negative pressure*, and is calculated using the following equation:

$$MI = \frac{P_r / f^{1/2}}{C_{MI}}$$

where P_r = peak rarefactional pressure, f = ultrasound frequency, and C_{MI} = 1 MPa/MHz.

▶ Baun J: *Ob/Gyn Sonography: An Illustrated Review*. Pasadena, CA, Davies Publishing, 2016, pp 440–441.

What is the purpose of using the Standard (formerly Universal) Precautions?

a. to reduce the risk of complications
b. to limit the risk of exposure to disease
c. to treat patients equally
d. to preserve patient confidentiality

Patient Care, Scanning Technique, and Physical Principles

A 470

B. To limit the risk of exposure to disease.

The Standard Precautions (formerly Universal Precautions) were introduced in the 1980s to limit healthcare workers' contact with patients' bodily fluids through the wearing of nonporous medical gloves, goggles, face shields, gowns, and other protective gear.

▶ Penny SM, Fox TB, Herring Godwin C: *Examination Review for Ultrasound: Sonographic Principles & Instrumentation*. Philadelphia, Lippincott Williams & Wilkins, 2011, ch 6.

471

Most infections that patients obtain from hospital stays can be reduced or eliminated by having patients and healthcare workers:

a. wash their hands
b. wear gloves
c. wear masks
d. wear gowns

Patient Care, Scanning Technique, and Physical Principles

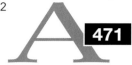

A. Wash their hands.

Proper hand washing is the most effective procedure for preventing the spread of disease.

▶ Penny SM, Fox TB, Herring Godwin C: *Examination Review for Ultrasound: Sonographic Principles & Instrumentation*. Philadelphia, Lippincott Williams & Wilkins, 2011, ch 6.

In a patient for whom it is necessary to take respiratory precautions, which of the following must be worn as part of patient care?

a. gloves
b. gown
c. cap
d. mask

Patient Care, Scanning Technique, and Physical Principles

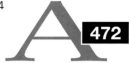

D. Mask.

A HEPA (high-efficiency particulate arrestance) filter mask must be worn by either the patient or the sonographer when performing ultrasound on a patient in respiratory isolation. These exams are usually performed in a negative pressure room specially designed for patients in respiratory isolation.

▶ Penny SM, Fox TB, Herring Godwin C: *Examination Review for Ultrasound: Sonographic Principles & Instrumentation.* Philadelphia, Lippincott Williams & Wilkins, 2011, ch 6.

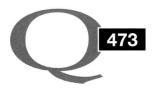

A patient with a possible placenta previa who is actively bleeding and near term should be scanned:

a. transabdominally only
b. in Fowler's position
c. transperineally
d. in Trendelenburg position

Patient Care, Scanning Technique, and Physical Principles

C. Transperineally.

Placing the transducer on the perineal area allows visualization of the cervix without entering the vagina and possibly causing more bleeding. Sometimes in such cases endovaginal sonography is clinically indicated, but *transperineal* (also known as *translabial*) scanning is safe and allows a close view of the cervical area.

▶ Gill KA: Introduction to diagnostic ultrasound. In Gill KA: *Ultrasound in Obstetrics and Gynecology: A Practitioner's Guide*. Pasadena, CA, Davies Publishing, 2014, p 16.

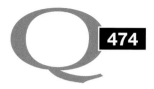 **474**

The transducer most suitable to visualizing a large leiomyoma in an obese patient is:

a. 3.5 MHz sector
b. 3.5 MHz curvilinear
c. 5.0 MHz sector
d. 5.0 MHz curvilinear

Patient Care, Scanning Technique, and Physical Principles

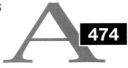

B. 3.5 MHz curvilinear.

The curvilinear array will allow a larger field of view. The lower frequency is necessary for greater depth of penetration.

- Baun J: *Ob/Gyn Sonography: An Illustrated Review*. Pasadena, CA, Davies Publishing, 2016, p 498.
- Gill KA: Introduction to diagnostic ultrasound. In Gill KA: *Ultrasound in Obstetrics and Gynecology: A Practitioner's Guide*. Pasadena, CA, Davies Publishing, 2014, pp 14, 15, 224.

949

Of the following, which is best for demonstrating bony structures when imaging in 3D?

a. surface rendering
b. minimum-intensity projections
c. multiplanar viewing
d. maximum-intensity projections

A 475

D. Maximum-intensity projections.

Surface rendering and minimum-intensity projections demonstrate soft tissues and organs, while the multiplanar images show longitudinal, transverse, and coronal planes separately.

▶ Bega G, Merton DA: Volume sonography. In Gill KA: *Ultrasound in Obstetrics and Gynecology: A Practitioner's Guide*. Pasadena, CA, Davies Publishing, 2014, p 415.

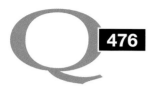

What type of transducer produced this image of an ovarian cyst?

a. sector
b. curved linear
c. phased array
d. linear

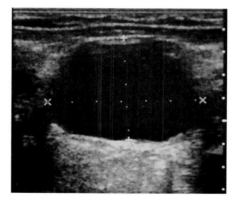

Patient Care, Scanning Technique, and Physical Principles

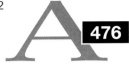

D. Linear.

Linear transducers produce images in a rectangular format. All of the other types produce triangular or wedge-shaped images.

- Baun J: *Ob/Gyn Sonography: An Illustrated Review*. Pasadena, CA, Davies Publishing, 2016, p 450.
- Gill KA: Introduction to diagnostic ultrasound. In Gill KA: *Ultrasound in Obstetrics and Gynecology: A Practitioner's Guide*. Pasadena, CA, Davies Publishing, 2014, p 11.

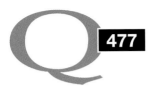

953

When one views a coronal endovaginal image of the uterus, the patient's left side will be seen at the:

a. right side of the image
b. top of the image
c. bottom of the image
d. left side of the image

Patient Care, Scanning Technique, and Physical Principles

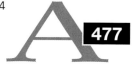

A. Right side of the image.

Transvaginal (endovaginal) coronal planes are analogous to the transverse transabdominal plane in that the left side of the image is the patient's right, and the right side of the image is the patient's left.

▶ Gill KA: Introduction to diagnostic ultrasound. In Gill KA: *Ultrasound in Obstetrics and Gynecology: A Practitioner's Guide*. Pasadena, CA, Davies Publishing, 2014, pp 18–19.

955

As you look at a longitudinal endovaginal image of a patient, the patient's feet would be toward:

a. the bottom of the image
b. the right side of the image
c. the left side of the image
d. the top of the image

Patient Care, Scanning Technique, and Physical Principles

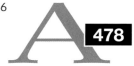

D. The top of the image.

Longitudinal transvaginal ultrasound images are viewed as if the patient has been imaged upside down. The top of the image is the patient's feet, the bottom of the image is the patient's head, the left side of the image is anterior, and the right side of the image is posterior.

▶ Gill KA: Introduction to diagnostic ultrasound. In Gill KA: *Ultrasound in Obstetrics and Gynecology: A Practitioner's Guide*. Pasadena, CA, Davies Publishing, 2014, p 19.

957

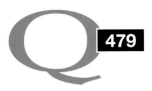

What is the name of an ultrasound probe constructed with the piezoelectric elements arranged in several parallel lines, permitting acquisition of two orthogonal planes of echo data simultaneously and used in 3D and 4D imaging?

a. linear array
b. convex array
c. matrix array
d. phased array

Patient Care, Scanning Technique, and Physical Principles

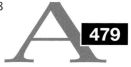

C. Matrix array.

The matrix array transducer, also called a 2D array transducer, looks like a phased array transducer but operates differently. Instead of acquiring information in one plane (1D), the probe acquires information in two planes simultaneously (2D). The matrix array transducer permits real-time 3D and 4D scanning without any moving parts.

▶ Baun J: *Ob/Gyn Sonography: An Illustrated Review*. Pasadena, CA, Davies Publishing, 2016, p 451.

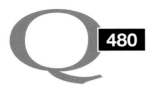

What is the name of an ultrasound probe constructed with the piezoelectric elements arranged in a short, compact linear configuration and fired using timing delays to create a wedge-shaped, or sector, image?

a. linear array
b. matrix array
c. phased array
d. convex array

A 480

C. Phased array.

In a phased array transducer, electrical impulses are sent to the piezoelectric elements with minute time differences in between, permitting for electronic steering and focusing of the beam. This type of transducer creates a sector- or vector-shaped image.

▶ Baun J: *Ob/Gyn Sonography: An Illustrated Review*. Pasadena, CA, Davies Publishing, 2016, p 451.

▶ Penny SM, Fox TB, Herring Godwin C: *Examination Review for Ultrasound: Sonographic Principles & Instrumentation*. Philadelphia, Lippincott Williams & Wilkins, 2011, ch 2.

481

Where should you place the cursors to measure the long axis of the cervix?

a. uterine isthmus to internal os
b. uterine isthmus to external os
c. internal os to external os
d. vaginal introitus to external os

Patient Care, Scanning Technique, and Physical Principles

481

C. Internal os to external os.

Cervical length is typically measured in long axis from the internal os to the external os. If any funneling is identified, the dimension of the funneling should be measured as well.

▶ Baun J: *Ob/Gyn Sonography: An Illustrated Review*. Pasadena, CA, Davies Publishing, 2016, pp 466–467.

963

Q 482

Which of the following is NOT a routine part of performing an endovaginal ultrasound exam?

a. explaining the nature and importance of the procedure to the patient
b. asking the patient to continue to maintain a full bladder
c. applying a protective sheath to the probe
d. applying generous amounts of lubricant to the probe

Patient Care, Scanning Technique, and Physical Principles

A 482

B. Asking the patient to continue to maintain a full bladder.

Endovaginal (transvaginal) ultrasound should be performed with an empty maternal urinary bladder. Ask the patient to empty just before performing the exam, especially if the patient had a full bladder for the first part of the exam.

▶ Baun J: *Ob/Gyn Sonography: An Illustrated Review*. Pasadena, CA, Davies Publishing, 2016, p 464.

The only Doppler ultrasound modality that permits the quantification of flow states with angle-corrected velocity measurements is:

a. pulsed-wave spectral Doppler
b. color Doppler imaging
c. power Doppler imaging
d. continuous-wave spectral Doppler

Patient Care, Scanning Technique, and Physical Principles

A 483

A. Pulsed-wave spectral Doppler.

Both continuous-wave (CW) spectral Doppler and pulsed-wave (PW) spectral Doppler permit measurement of flow velocities, but only PW spectral Doppler permits angle-corrected flow velocities, allowing for more accurate measurement of velocities. With CW Doppler, a zero-degree angle is assumed. Color and power Doppler permit visualization of flow but not quantification.

▶ Baun J: *Ob/Gyn Sonography: An Illustrated Review*. Pasadena, CA, Davies Publishing, 2016, p 448.

In this image of the lower uterine segment, what is the reason for nonvisualization of the cervix?

a. Shadowing from the lower uterus is obscuring the cervix.

b. The transducer is backward.

c. The bladder is too full.

d. Fetal parts are in the way.

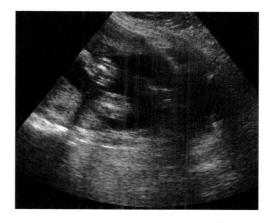

Patient Care, Scanning Technique, and Physical Principles

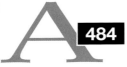

A. Shadowing from the lower uterus is obscuring the cervix.

This transabdominal image of the lower uterine segment is taken after the patient has emptied her bladder, which is appropriate, as a full bladder can artificially lengthen a cervix or mask cervical dilatation. However, the cervix is not adequately visualized here. The reason is that the curvature of the uterus is causing a shadow that is obscuring the cervix. Changing the angle of insonation or performing a transvaginal ultrasound exam will correct this problem.

- Baun J: *Ob/Gyn Sonography: An Illustrated Review*. Pasadena, CA, Davies Publishing, 2016, p 452.
- Gill KA: *Ultrasound in Obstetrics and Gynecology: A Practitioner's Guide*. Pasadena, CA, Davies Publishing, 2014, pp 7, 452.

The split-image artifact can be eliminated by:

a. having the patient take in a deep breath
b. changing the frequency of the transducer
c. changing the focus of the transducer
d. scanning from a different projection

Patient Care, Scanning Technique, and Physical Principles

D. Scanning from a different projection.

A split-image or ghost artifact is a refraction artifact caused by the rectus abdominis muscles. With this artifact a duplicate "ghost" image is placed alongside the real image. Scanning from a different angle will eliminate this artifact.

▶ Baun J: *Ob/Gyn Sonography: An Illustrated Review*. Pasadena, CA, Davies Publishing, 2016, p 454.

▶ Gill KA: Introduction to diagnostic ultrasound. In Gill KA: *Ultrasound in Obstetrics and Gynecology: A Practitioner's Guide*. Pasadena, CA, Davies Publishing, 2014, p 8.

# 486

A patient presents for a pelvic sonogram post dilatation and curettage. Within the uterine cavity there are several bright focal reflectors with lower-level echoes emanating from behind each one. This artifact is referred to as:

a. comet-tail
b. ring-down
c. mirror-image
d. side-lobe

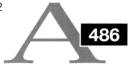

B. Ring-down.

Ring-down artifact is seen deep to foci of air. Its appearance is similar to that of *reverberation* (parallel linear echoes) but with ring-down artifact the echoes are very small and caused by the vibration of the air molecules.

- Kremkau FW: *Sonography: Principles and Instruments*, 8th edition. St. Louis, Elsevier, 2011, pp 180–181.
- Kremkau FW: Artifacts in scanning. In Hagen-Ansert SL (ed): *Textbook of Diagnostic Sonography*, 7th edition. St. Louis, Elsevier Mosby, p 99.
- Merritt CRB: Physics of ultrasound. In Rumack CM (ed): *Diagnostic Ultrasound*, 4th edition. St. Louis, Mosby, 2011, pp 2–33.

To what is the arrow in this image pointing?

a. refractive shadowing
b. slice-thickness artifact
c. posterior enhancement
d. ring-down artifact

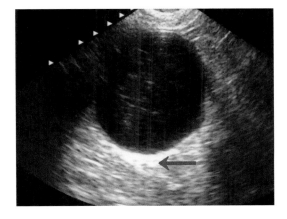

Patient Care, Scanning Technique, and Physical Principles / AIT—Hotspot

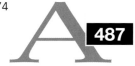

C. Posterior enhancement.

Posterior enhancement, previously called "through transmission," is demonstrated by increased echogenicity (echoes that are brighter than surrounding echoes) behind a fluid-containing structure.

- Baun J: *Ob/Gyn Sonography: An Illustrated Review*. Pasadena, CA, Davies Publishing, 2016, p 452.
- Gill KA: Introduction to diagnostic ultrasound. In Gill KA: *Ultrasound in Obstetrics and Gynecology: A Practitioner's Guide*. Pasadena, CA, Davies Publishing, 2014, pp 6, 7.

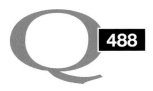

What artifact appears as equally spaced, bright linear echoes resulting from repeated reflections from specular-type interfaces?

a. refractions
b. section thickness
c. side lobes
d. reverberation

Patient Care, Scanning Technique, and Physical Principles

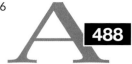

D. Reverberation.

Reverberation appears as parallel or concentric linear echoes, decreasing in brightness with depth, which is caused by the sound bouncing back and forth between strong specular reflectors.

▶ Baun J: *Ob/Gyn Sonography: An Illustrated Review*. Pasadena, CA, Davies Publishing, 2016, pp 452–453.

489

What artifact results from the reduction in amplitude of echoes lying deep to a highly reflective interface?

a. posterior acoustic enhancement
b. posterior acoustic shadowing
c. section-thickness artifact
d. mirror-image artifact

Patient Care, Scanning Technique, and Physical Principles

A 489

B. Posterior acoustic shadowing.

Shadowing occurs when sound travels through an area of increased attenuation. Structures that are highly reflective, like air or bone, will have shadowing deep to them because there are no echoes to return to the transducer.

▶ Baun J: *Ob/Gyn Sonography: An Illustrated Review*. Pasadena, CA, Davies Publishing, 2016, p 452.

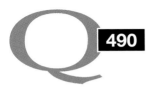

Which sonographic modality displays a single B-mode line of site along a horizontal axis?

a. M-mode
b. B-mode
c. pulsed-wave Doppler
d. B-color

Patient Care, Scanning Technique, and Physical Principles

490

A. M-mode.

M-mode, which stands for "motion mode," displays a single scan line of information over time. It is used for documenting movement, such as that of the fetal heart. It is a form of *B-mode* (*brightness mode*), not Doppler. *B-color* is colorization of B-mode pixels.

▶ Baun J: *Ob/Gyn Sonography: An Illustrated Review*. Pasadena, CA, Davies Publishing, 2016, p 444.

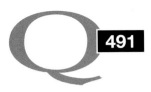

What is the term for the two-dimensional sonographic method of displaying the amplitude of a returning echo as a shade of gray?

a. B-mode
b. real time
c. static scanning
d. M-mode

Patient Care, Scanning Technique, and Physical Principles

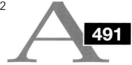

A. B-mode.

B-mode stands for *brightness mode*. Echo amplitude is displayed as a shade of gray, from black to white. *M-mode* (*motion mode*) is a type of B-mode that examines a single scan line. *Real-time* and *static* scanning are two ways of obtaining B-mode information; static scanning is obsolete.

▶ Baun J: *Ob/Gyn Sonography: An Illustrated Review*. Pasadena, CA, Davies Publishing, 2016, pp 442–443.

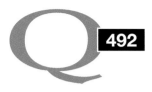

Ultrasound frequencies returning to the transducer that are generated by shifts in phase and frequency within the tissue itself are called:

a. fundamental
b. harmonic
c. secondary
d. tertiary

Patient Care, Scanning Technique, and Physical Principles

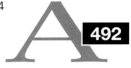

B. Harmonic.

Vibrations in the tissue caused by the incident sound create sound waves that return to the transducer, called *harmonics*. These harmonic signals have frequencies that are multiples of the incident, or fundamental, frequency. When *tissue harmonic imaging* (THI) is used, the second harmonic is used, which is double the fundamental frequency.

▶ Baun J: *Ob/Gyn Sonography: An Illustrated Review*. Pasadena, CA, Davies Publishing, 2016, p 449.

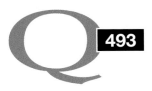

493

The B-mode method of generating, processing, and combining several image subframes into a single frame is called:

a. compounding
b. harmonics
c. enhancement
d. digital signal processing

Patient Care, Scanning Technique, and Physical Principles

A. Compounding.

Spatial compounding, which goes by many trade names depending on the manufacturer, permits visualization of a structure from multiple directions, reducing artifacts such as edge shadowing and decreasing a type of noise called *acoustic speckle*.

▶ Baun J: *Ob/Gyn Sonography: An Illustrated Review*. Pasadena, CA, Davies Publishing, 2016, p 442.

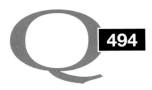

494

How much urine must be retained in the bladder for transabdominal sonography?

a. 200 cc
b. 300 cc
c. 400 cc
d. 500 cc

Patient Care, Scanning Technique, and Physical Principles

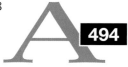

D. 500 cc.

Approximately 500 cc of fluid or more is needed in the urinary bladder for adequate visualization of pelvic structures. Generally, the patient is asked to finish drinking 32 ounces of water at least 45 minutes before the start of the exam, assuming that the patient is not dehydrated beforehand.

▶ Baun J: *Ob/Gyn Sonography: An Illustrated Review*. Pasadena, CA, Davies Publishing, 2016, p 463.

Doppler information is obtained from analyzing and displaying:

a. Rayleigh backscatter
b. specular reflectors
c. nonspecular reflectors
d. transmitted energy

Patient Care, Scanning Technique, and Physical Principles

A 495

A. Rayleigh backscatter.

Red blood cells are a specific type of nonspecular reflector called a *Rayleigh scatterer*. Rayleigh scatterers are very small in relation to the wavelength of the incident beam.

▶ Baun J: *Ob/Gyn Sonography: An Illustrated Review*. Pasadena, CA, Davies Publishing, 2016, p 446.

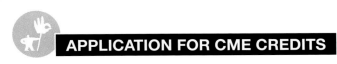

APPLICATION FOR CME CREDITS

ScoreCards™
for Ob/Gyn Sonography

This continuing medical educational (CME) activity is approved for 12 hours of credit by the Society of Diagnostic Medical Sonography. This credit may be applied as follows:

- Sonographers and technologists may apply these hours toward the CME requirements of the ARDMS, ARRT, and/or CCI, as well as to the CME requirements of most other organizations that may accredit your facility.

- SDMS-approved credit is not applicable toward the AMA Physician's Recognition Award but may be applicable to the CME requirements for physicians associated with accredited ultrasound facilities. Be sure to confirm requirements with the pertinent organizations.

- If you have any questions whatsoever about CME requirements that affect you, please contact the responsible organization directly for current information. CME requirements can and sometimes do change.

Objectives of This Activity

Upon completion of this educational activity, you will be able to:

1. Identify normal and abnormal fetal and female pelvic anatomy and physiology.
2. Describe how, when, and why ultrasonography is applied in the practice of obstetrics and gynecology.
3. Differentiate between normal and abnormal obstetric and gynecologic sonographic findings.
4. Explain the correlations between these findings and pertinent laboratory and imaging studies.
5. Describe how, when, and why fetal and gynecologic measurements are made.

How to Obtain CME Credit

To apply for credit, please do all of the following:

1. Read and study the cards and complete the interactive exercises they contain.
2. Photocopy and complete the following applicant information page, evaluation questionnaire (you grade us!), and CME answer sheet.

CME Application   993

3. Return the completed forms together with payment of the administrative and processing fee of $39.50 (if you are the book's original purchaser) or $49.50 (for borrowers) to the following address.

Davies Publishing, Inc.
CME Coordinator
32 South Raymond Avenue, Suite 4
Pasadena, California 91105-1961

You can also fax the appropriate pages to 626-792-5308 and pay by credit card. We grade quizzes within 24 business hours of receipt and will email your certificate to the email address you provide in your application form. Questions? Please call us at 626-792-3046.

4. If more than one person will be applying for credit, be sure to photocopy the applicant information, evaluation form, and CME quiz so that you always have the original on hand for use.

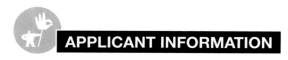

APPLICANT INFORMATION

ScoreCards for Ob/Gyn Sonography

Name _____ Date of Birth _____

Your degrees and credentials _____

Address _____

City/State/Zip _____

Telephone _____ Email (required) _____

ARDMS# _____ ARRT# _____ SDMS# _____ CCI # _____

Credit Card # _____ Exp Date _____ 3- or 4-digit code _____

Name and address on credit card (if different)

_____

❏ I purchased this book myself.   ❏ I borrowed the book.

Signature and date certifying your completion of the activity

_____

NOTE

The original purchaser of this CME activity is entitled to submit this CME application for an administrative fee of $39.50. Please enclose a check payable to Davies Publishing, Inc., or include credit card information with your application. Others may also submit applications for CME credits by completing the activity for an administrative fee of $49.50. The CME administrative fee helps to defray the cost of processing, evaluating, and maintaining a record of your application and the credit you earn. Fees may change without notice. For the current fee, call us at 626-792-3046, email us at cme@daviespublishing.com, or write to us at the aforementioned address. We will be happy to help!

Evaluation—You Grade Us!

Please let us know what you think of the *ScoreCards* study system. Participating in this quality survey is a requirement for CME applicants, and it benefits future readers by ensuring that current readers are satisfied and, if not, that their comments and opinions are heard and taken into account.

1 Why did you purchase *ScoreCards*? (Circle your primary reason.)

Registry review   Course text   Clinical reference   CME activity

2 Have you used *ScoreCards* for other reasons, too? (Circle all that apply.)

Registry review   Course text   Clinical reference   CME activity

3 To what extent did *ScoreCards* meet its stated objectives and your needs? (Circle one.)

Greatly   Moderately   Minimally   Insignificantly

4 The content of *ScoreCards* was (circle one):

Just right   Too basic   Too advanced

5 The quality of the questions, explanations, illustrations, and case examples was mainly (circle one):

Excellent   Good   Fair   Poor

6 The manner in which *ScoreCards* presents the material is mainly (circle one):

Excellent   Good   Fair   Poor

7 If you used *ScoreCards* to prepare for the registry exam, did you also use other materials or take any exam-preparation courses?

No   Yes (please specify what materials and courses)

_____

_____

8 If you used *ScoreCards* for a course, please list the course name, the instructor's name, the name of the school or program, and any other textbooks you may have used:

Course/Instructor/School or program _____

_____

CME Application   997

9 What did you like best about *ScoreCards*?

_____

_____

10 What did you like least about *ScoreCards*?

_____

_____

11 If you used *ScoreCards* to prepare for your registry exam in vascular technology, did you pass?

   Yes   No   Haven't yet taken it

12 May we quote any of your comments in our catalogs or promotional material?

   Yes   No   Further comment

_____

_____

_____

ANSWER SHEET

ScoreCards for Ob/Gyn Sonography

1. a b c d	21. a b c d	41. a b c d	61. a b c d	81. a b c d	101. a b c d
2. a b c d	22. a b c d	42. a b c d	62. a b c d	82. a b c d	102. a b c d
3. a b c d	23. a b c d	43. a b c d	63. a b c d	83. a b c d	103. a b c d
4. a b c d	24. a b c d	44. a b c d	64. a b c d	84. a b c d	104. a b c d
5. a b c d	25. a b c d	45. a b c d	65. a b c d	85. a b c d	105. a b c d
6. a b c d	26. a b c d	46. a b c d	66. a b c d	86. a b c d	106. a b c d
7. a b c d	27. a b c d	47. a b c d	67. a b c d	87. a b c d	107. a b c d
8. a b c d	28. a b c d	48. a b c d	68. a b c d	88. a b c d	108. a b c d
9. a b c d	29. a b c d	49. a b c d	69. a b c d	89. a b c d	109. a b c d
10. a b c d	30. a b c d	50. a b c d	70. a b c d	90. a b c d	110. a b c d
11. a b c d	31. a b c d	51. a b c d	71. a b c d	91. a b c d	111. a b c d
12. a b c d	32. a b c d	52. a b c d	72. a b c d	92. a b c d	112. a b c d
13. a b c d	33. a b c d	53. a b c d	73. a b c d	93. a b c d	113. a b c d
14. a b c d	34. a b c d	54. a b c d	74. a b c d	94. a b c d	114. a b c d
15. a b c d	35. a b c d	55. a b c d	75. a b c d	95. a b c d	115. a b c d
16. a b c d	36. a b c d	56. a b c d	76. a b c d	96. a b c d	116. a b c d
17. a b c d	37. a b c d	57. a b c d	77. a b c d	97. a b c d	117. a b c d
18. a b c d	38. a b c d	58. a b c d	78. a b c d	98. a b c d	118. a b c d
19. a b c d	39. a b c d	59. a b c d	79. a b c d	99. a b c d	119. a b c d
20. a b c d	40. a b c d	60. a b c d	80. a b c d	100. a b c d	120. a b c d

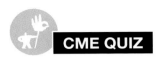

CME QUIZ

ScoreCards for Ob/Gyn Sonography

Please answer the following questions after you have completed the CME activity. There is one best answer for each question. Circle it on the answer sheet on the preceding page. Passing criterion is 70%. Applicants will have no more than 3 attempts to pass.

1. In a premenarcheal patient, what is the term for an accumulation of fluid in the vagina but not the uterus?
   a. hematometrocolpos
   b. hydrocolpos
   c. hematometra
   d. hydrometra

2. In the first trimester, what does the sonographic identification of cervical dilatation suggest?
   a. spontaneous abortion
   b. incomplete abortion
   c. threatened abortion
   d. inevitable abortion

3. Color Doppler imaging may be used to evaluate:
   a. peak systolic and end-diastolic velocities
   b. resistivity indices

1000 CME Application

    c. pulsatility indices
    d. presence of flow

4. Which of the following actions can both hospital workers and patients take to reduce or eliminate most infections that patients can contract during a hospital stay?
    a. wearing gloves
    b. wearing masks
    c. washing their hands
    d. wearing gowns

5. Where should you place the spectral range gate (sample volume) when performing a Doppler study of the uterine artery?
    a. near its origin at the internal iliac artery
    b. near the cervix
    c. mid-vessel, with strongest color signal
    d. anywhere along its course

6. The condition characterized by the deep invasion of placental villi into the myometrium but not the serosal layer is called:
    a. placenta percreta
    b. chorioangioma
    c. placenta increta
    d. placental abruption

7. Which sonographic modality displays a single B-mode line of site along a horizontal axis?
   a. B-mode
   b. pulsed-wave Doppler
   c. B-color
   d. M-mode

8. Which of the following will demonstrate reversal of flow in the presence of tricuspid regurgitation?
   a. umbilical artery
   b. middle cerebral artery
   c. ductus venosus
   d. ductus arteriosus

9. To obtain a biparietal measurement, which plane of section through the fetal head should you use?
   a. sagittal
   b. transaxial
   c. occipital
   d. cephalic

10. A mass of endometrial tissue projecting out from the surface of the endometrium and into the endometrial cavity is:
    a. an endometrial carcinoma
    b. a fibroid
    c. an endometrial polyp
    d. an adhesion

1002   CME Application

11. What is the approximate crown-rump length at the time embryonic cardiac activity can first be visualized?
    a. 2–4 mm
    b. 1–3 mm
    c. 3–5 mm
    d. 4–6 mm

12. In which portion of the fallopian tube does fertilization usually occur?
    a. interstitial
    b. cornua
    c. ampulla
    d. fimbrium

13. What effect does maternal diabetes have on the fetal abdominal circumference (AC)?
    a. Diabetes makes the stomach dilate, causing an enlarged AC.
    b. Diabetes makes the AC smaller than normal due to malnutrition.
    c. Diabetes makes the amount of fetal body fat increase, causing an enlarged AC.
    d. Diabetes makes the intestines swell, causing an enlarged AC.

14. The sonographic appearance of the fetal forearm in the anatomic position normally demonstrates that:
    a. the ulna is longer than the radius proximally
    b. the ulna is positioned lateral to the radius
    c. the ulna is on the same side as the thumb
    d. B and C

CME Application   1003

15. Which of these measurements represents a normal value for nuchal translucency?
    a. <3.5 mm
    b. <4.5 mm
    c. <5.5 mm
    d. <2.5 mm

16. The most common vascular abnormality of the umbilical cord is:
    a. four-vessel cord
    b. cord cyst
    c. single umbilical artery (SUA)
    d. short cord

17. All of the following are used to treat infertility patients EXCEPT:
    a. clomiphene citrate
    b. human chorionic gonadotropin
    c. metformin
    d. methotrexate

18. What would be the most suitable transducer for visualizing a large leiomyoma in an
    obese patient?
    a. 3.5 MHz sector
    b. 5.0 MHz sector
    c. 3.5 MHz curvilinear
    d. 5.0 MHz curvilinear

1004   CME Application

19. Your patient presents with a positive beta-hCG titer and shoulder pain. Ultrasound demonstrates an empty uterus, free fluid in the cul-de-sac, and ascites in Morison's pouch. You suspect:
    a. ruptured ectopic pregnancy
    b. hydronephrosis
    c. gallbladder stones
    d. pericardial effusion

20. A fetal head shape corresponding to a cephalic index of 64% is termed:
    a. brachycephaly
    b. cloverleaf skull
    c. strawberry skull
    d. dolichocephaly

21. You want to determine the date of your patient's last menstrual period. Which is the best question to ask?
    a. What is your LMP?
    b. Do you know when your last menstrual period was?
    c. When was the last day of your last menstrual period?
    d. When was the first day of your last menstrual period?

22. Which of the following can cause female pseudohermaphroditism?
    a. low levels of androgens
    b. congenital adrenal hyperplasia
    c. decreased progesterone production
    d. DES exposure

23. Color Doppler imaging confirms the presence of umbilical cord between the fetal presenting part and the internal cervical os. This is termed:
    a. vasa previa
    b. battledore placenta
    c. nuchal cord
    d. velamentous insertion

24. Which procedure performed at the internal cervical os requires a cesarean section at delivery?
    a. McDonald's procedure
    b. Valsalva maneuver
    c. transabdominal cerclage
    d. digital examination

25. One indication of an abnormal pregnancy would be:
    a. an embryo with a calcified yolk sac
    b. a defined double decidual ring around the intrauterine gestational sac
    c. a round or oval gestational sac within the uterus
    d. the double sac sign within an intrauterine gestational sac

26. The term *heterotopic pregnancy* means:
    a. an irregular sac-like structure in the endometrium
    b. a simultaneous intra- and extrauterine pregnancy
    c. an irregular sac-like structure in the adnexa
    d. an abdominal pregnancy

1006   CME Application

27. What should your measurement of femur length include?
    a. femoral head
    b. condyles
    c. epiphysis
    d. diaphysis

28. What is the blood test that might indicate that a patient's ovarian cancer has returned?
    a. CA-125
    b. beta-hCG
    c. FSH
    d. TSH

29. What condition is suggested by an enlarged ovary with a rounded shape and peripherally located follicles in a "string of pearls" configuration?
    a. theca-lutein cysts
    b. Stein-Leventhal syndrome
    c. hemorrhagic cysts
    d. ovarian hyperstimulation syndrome

30. Of the following cranial structures, which is the landmark for locating the atria of the lateral ventricles?
    a. choroid plexus
    b. cavum septi pellucidi
    c. corpus callosum
    d. cisterna magna

31. Approximately when are the ossification centers of the fetal spine sonographically visible?
    a. 10 weeks
    b. 18 weeks
    c. 16 weeks
    d. 22 weeks

32. What is the term for the presence of an accessory fragment of lung with no connection to the tracheobronchial tree and with a separate systemic arterial circulation?
    a. pulmonary sequestration
    b. congenital pulmonary airway malformation
    c. diaphragmatic hernia
    d. diaphragmatic eventration

33. What is the name for the structural and developmental fetal abnormalities that occur in the presence of a chronic absence of amniotic fluid in a severely oligohydramniotic sac?
    a. Potter sequence
    b. bilateral renal agenesis
    c. Beckwith-Wiedemann syndrome
    d. Zellweger syndrome

34. An accessory lobe of the placenta located apart from the main placental body is called:
    a. circumvallate
    b. succenturiate
    c. circummarginate
    d. annular

35. Which fetal organ should you document if cystic fibrosis is suspected?
    a. spleen
    b. diaphragm
    c. gallbladder
    d. right kidney

36. Excessive accumulation of fluid in at least two fetal anatomic locations is called:
    a. anasarca
    b. ascites
    c. hydrops fetalis
    d. hydrocephalus

37. The uterus and fallopian tubes can be visualized using which of these invasive tests?
    a. intravenous pyelogram
    b. angiogram
    c. myelogram
    d. hysterosalpingogram

38. In the presence of pelvic inflammatory disease, what is the term for an inflammatory mass extending beyond the fallopian tubes?
    a. pyosalpinx
    b. hydrosalpinx
    c. tubo-ovarian abscess
    d. tubal carcinoma

39. A placenta with a few scattered bright echoes, slight indentations at the chorionic plate, and an unchanged basal layer is consistent with:
    a. grade 0 placenta
    b. grade I placenta
    c. grade II placenta
    d. grade III placenta

40. Precocious puberty may be associated with which of the following feminizing tumors?
    a. teratoma
    b. granulosa cell tumor
    c. serous cystadenoma
    d. arrhenoblastoma

41. What uterine form will result if the müllerian ducts completely fail to fuse?
    a. uterus didelphys
    b. septate uterus
    c. bicornuate uterus
    d. arcuate uterus

42. If a currently nonpregnant patient is G3P2102, how many preterm births has the patient had?
    a. 3
    b. 2
    c. 1
    d. none

1010   CME Application

43. Which procedure is used to treat massive polyhydramnios?
    a. percutaneous umbilical blood sampling
    b. pleuroamniotic shunting
    c. intrapartum amniotransfusion
    d. therapeutic amnioreduction

44. A placenta in which a loose chorionic membrane folds back upon itself and encircles the fetal surface is called:
    a. circummarginate
    b. succenturiate
    c. circumvallate
    d. annular

45. Which is a normal range for nuchal translucency measured between the 11th and 14th menstrual weeks?
    a. 1.0–4.0 mm
    b. 1.5–3.5 mm
    c. 1.0–3.0 mm
    d. 1.0–2.5 mm

46. Macroglossia is commonly associated with:
    a. Beckwith-Wiedemann syndrome
    b. trisomy 13
    c. maternal phenylketonuria (PKU)
    d. Treacher Collins syndrome

47. The longest portion of the fallopian tube is the:
    a. isthmus
    b. infundibulum
    c. ampulla
    d. interstitial portion

48. Normal nuchal fold thickness should not measure more than:
    a. 2–3 mm
    b. 3–4 mm
    c. 5–6 mm
    d. 4–5 mm

49. In which clinically serious condition do velamentously inserted cord vessels precede the fetal presenting part?
    a. vasa previa
    b. complete previa
    c. partial previa
    d. prolapsed cord

50. Which of these ligaments is the primary supporting ligament of the uterus, arising from the lateral aspect of the cervix and uterus and inserting along the lateral pelvic wall?
    a. round ligament
    b. broad ligament
    c. cardinal ligament
    d. uterosacral ligament

1012   CME Application

51. Which nonpelvic structure(s) should be scanned in the presence of a large leiomyoma?
    a. liver
    b. peritoneal cavity
    c. kidneys
    d. aorta

52. Which structure actively secretes human chorionic gonadotropin?
    a. ovary
    b. trophoblastic tissue
    c. pituitary gland
    d. adrenal gland

53. In the presence of endometrial fluid, how should you measure the endometrium?
    a. The entire thickness should be measured, including the hypoechoic border.
    b. From anterior basal layer to posterior basal layer, including the fluid.
    c. From anterior basal layer to the fluid, and from posterior basal layer to the fluid.
    d. Only the fluid is measured.

54. Polyhydramnios would be indicated by which of these single-deepest-pocket amniotic fluid measurements?
    a. >12 cm
    b. >14 cm
    c. >16 cm
    d. >8 cm

55. When is chorionic villus sampling (CVS) best performed?
    a. 4–6 weeks
    b. 14–16 weeks
    c. 10–13 weeks
    d. 16–18 weeks

56. Which of these sites is the most common for an ectopic pregnancy?
    a. cornua
    b. cervix
    c. abdomen
    d. ampulla

57. Physiologic herniation of the fetal midgut usually resolves by:
    a. 6 weeks
    b. 12 weeks
    c. 18 weeks
    d. 26 weeks

58. Which of the following abnormal congenital chromosomal conditions is usually accompanied by cystic hygroma?
    a. trisomy 13
    b. trisomy 21
    c. Treacher Collins syndrome
    d. Turner syndrome

1014   CME Application

59. Which of these fetal abnormalities may be associated with an abnormal decrease in maternal serum alpha-fetoprotein (MSAFP)?
   a. spina bifida
   b. omphalocele
   c. trisomy 21
   d. multiple gestations

60. A normal postmenopausal endometrium usually has a double-thickness measurement of:
   a. 5–7 mm
   b. 6–8 mm
   c. <5 mm
   d. >5 mm

61. An amniotic fluid index (AFI) is acquired by:
   a. subjective analysis
   b. summation of the measurement of two horizontal pockets
   c. measurement of the single deepest pocket
   d. summation of the measurements of the single deepest pocket in each uterine quadrant free of fetal parts

62. A fetal pole with cardiac motion should always be identifiable with transvaginal ultrasound by the time the mean sac diameter (MSD) measures:
   a. 16 mm
   b. 11 mm
   c. 22 mm
   d. 30 mm

63. An elevated level of maternal serum alpha-fetoprotein (MSAFP) would be associated with:
    a. omphalocele
    b. congenital diaphragmatic hernia
    c. umbilical vein varix
    d. gastroschisis

64. Which fetal anomaly is most specifically associated with maternal diabetes mellitus?
    a. caudal regression syndrome
    b. prune belly syndrome
    c. amniotic band sequence
    d. clinodactyly

65. After fetal demise, gas may appear in the fetal chest and/or abdomen resulting from tissue breakdown. What is this called?
    a. Spalding's sign
    b. Robert's sign
    c. Murphy's sign
    d. Deuel's sign

66. For performance of transvaginal ultrasound of the pelvis, visualization is enhanced with the bladder:
    a. completely empty
    b. completely full
    c. partially full
    d. as full as the patient can maintain during the course of the examination

1016   CME Application

67. A third trimester patient feels faint and nauseated during a sonographic study. These symptoms are probably caused by:
    a. eating prior to the study
    b. supine hypotensive syndrome
    c. rapid ingestion of fluids
    d. lying on her left side

68. Measurement of which hormone forms the basis for all current laboratory pregnancy tests?
    a. progesterone
    b. beta-hCG
    c. estradiol
    d. luteinizing hormone

69. You are estimating the menstrual age of a dolichocephalic fetus. What measurement would be best?
    a. biparietal diameter
    b. cephalic index
    c. head circumference
    d. BPD/AC ratio

70. What is the maximum normal anteroposterior (AP) thickness of a full-term placenta?
    a. 3 cm
    b. 4 cm
    c. 5 cm
    d. 6 cm

71. What structure is released from the ovary at ovulation?
    a. primary follicle
    b. secondary follicle
    c. dominant follicle
    d. ovum

72. Which of the following is the best definition of *tenting*?
    a. proliferation of placental tissue between the amnions in a twin pregnancy
    b. discoloration of amniotic fluid when blue dye is introduced
    c. use of a stent with a triangular tip
    d. elevation of the amnion by a needle when the membranes have not fused

73. Which of the following is associated with "stuck twin" syndrome?
    a. conjoined twins
    b. twin reversed arterial perfusion (TRAP)
    c. twin-to-twin transfusion syndrome (TTTS)
    d. vanishing twin

74. What term denotes premature separation of the placenta from the myometrium?
    a. placental abruption
    b. placenta previa
    c. placenta percreta
    d. placenta accreta

1018   CME Application

75. Abnormal shortening of the humerus is known as:
    a. micromelia
    b. mesomelia
    c. rhizomelia
    d. amelia

76. How far from the internal cervical os should the placental edge be located to indicate
    that the mother is NOT at increased risk for complications during delivery?
    a. ≥1.0 cm
    b. ≥1.5 cm
    c. ≥2.5 cm
    d. ≥2.0 cm

77. What is the best method for visualizing endometrial polyps?
    a. laparoscopy
    b. hysterosonography
    c. transvaginal sonography
    d. full-bladder transabdominal sonography

78. With endovaginal sonography, how early can a gestational sac can be demonstrated?
    a. 4–5 menstrual weeks
    b. 2–3 menstrual weeks
    c. 5–6 menstrual weeks
    d. 6–7 menstrual weeks

79. What is the name for a vascular tumor of the chorion?
    a. angioma
    b. chorioangioma
    c. hemangioma
    d. angiomyoma

80. The reduction in amplitude of echoes lying deep to a highly reflective interface produces which artifact?
    a. posterior acoustic enhancement
    b. section thickness
    c. mirror image
    d. posterior acoustic shadowing

81. The most common and accurate method of assessing fetal lung maturity is:
    a. placental grading
    b. comparing fetal lung to liver echogenicity
    c. presence of fetal breathing movements
    d. amniocentesis

82. A follicle that does not rupture and release the ovum forms what type of cyst?
    a. theca-lutein cyst
    b. cystadenoma
    c. follicular cyst
    d. cystic teratoma

1020   CME Application

83. An 18-week ultrasound demonstrates that the fetus is missing a hand. The most likely diagnosis is:
    a. amniotic band sequence
    b. failure of amnion-chorion fusion
    c. limb–body wall complex
    d. Arnold-Chiari malformation

84. The condition in which at least three of these anomalies—vertebral defects, anal atresia, cardiac defects, tracheoesophageal fistula, renal anomalies, and limb abnormalities—occur in the same fetus is called:
    a. VACTERL association
    b. Ellis–van Creveld syndrome
    c. Holt-Oram syndrome
    d. Meckel-Gruber syndrome

85. Up to 10 weeks, the most accurate measurement of gestational age is:
    a. biparietal diameter
    b. mean sac diameter
    c. yolk sac size
    d. crown-rump length

86. When does regression of the corpus luteum cyst of pregnancy typically occur?
    a. 6–8 weeks
    b. 12–16 weeks

c. 8–10 weeks
d. 10–12 weeks

87. Both parents have the same autosomal recessive disorder. What is the probability that they will pass it on to their offspring?
   a. 100%
   b. 75%
   c. 50%
   d. 25%

88. Which type of congenital diaphragmatic hernia is most common?
   a. left-sided hernia
   b. right-sided hernia
   c. bilateral hernias
   d. A and B with equal frequency

89. Until about what menstrual age is the fetal transcerebellar diameter in millimeters equivalent to fetal menstrual age in weeks?
   a. 12 weeks
   b. 15 weeks
   c. 24 weeks
   d. 20 weeks

1022   CME Application

90. Three days after undergoing cesarean section, a febrile patient presents for pelvic ultrasound, which reveals echogenic and anechoic areas within the endometrial cavity. These findings are most consistent with:
    a. adenomyosis
    b. bladder flap hematoma
    c. retained products of conception
    d. retained intrauterine contraceptive device

91. Which uterine position is most commonly visualized when the urinary bladder is empty?
    a. anteverted
    b. anteflexed
    c. retroverted
    d. retroflexed

92. Decreased hormonal production during menopause results in:
    a. decreased cervical mucus
    b. increased irregular bleeding
    c. enlargement of fibroids
    d. breast enlargement

93. The uterine artery arises from the internal iliac artery and anastomoses with:
    a. a branch of the ovarian artery
    b. the external iliac artery
    c. the common iliac artery
    d. the arcuate arteries

94. As the uterus prepares for the implantation of a conceptus toward menstruation, how do cyclic changes in hormone levels affect hemodynamics in the uterine arteries?
    a. Uterine artery pulsatility increases.
    b. Uterine artery resistance increases.
    c. Uterine artery resistance decreases.
    d. There is no discernible change in blood flow.

95. Estrogen during pregnancy affects coexisting fibroids by:
    a. causing fibroid growth
    b. slowing the growth of fibroids
    c. causing degeneration of fibroids
    d. causing additional fibroids to form

96. What is the name of the outer glandular portion of the ovary that contains the follicles?
    a. medulla
    b. transitional zone
    c. cortex
    d. mesovarium

97. What potential trisomy 21 marker may be measured in the first trimester with or without a nuchal translucency measurement?
    a. nasal bone
    b. liver length
    c. middle phalanx of the fifth digit
    d. foot length

1024   CME Application

98. What is the term for the position of a fetus with the feet presenting?
    a. complete breech
    b. footling breech
    c. cephalic
    d. frank breech

99. What is the name of the potential space between the anterior bladder surface and the anterior abdominal wall?
    a. space of Retzius
    b. fornix
    c. pouch of Douglas
    d. cul-de-sac

100. In a fetus with spina bifida, the sonographic appearance of a compressed cerebellum that obliterates the region of the cisterna magna and distorts the head shape is known as the:
    a. lemon sign
    b. banana sign
    c. strawberry sign
    d. pear sign

101. The neonatal ovary normally has a volume of:
    a. ≤1.0 cc
    b. 2–3 cc
    c. 3–4 cc
    d. ≥1.0 cc

102. What is the normal sonographic appearance of fetal bowel echogenicity?
    a. less echogenic than bone and more echogenic than liver
    b. more echogenic than bone and less echogenic than liver
    c. more echogenic than liver and less echogenic than spleen
    d. more echogenic than spleen and isoechoic with liver

103. Of the following statements which is MOST true for ovarian tumors?
    a. benign
    b. metastatic
    c. solid
    d. mixed solid/cystic

104. Which of the following methods is best for differentiating a leiomyoma from focal uterine contractions?
    a. Examine using spectral Doppler.
    b. Reevaluate after 30 minutes.
    c. Have the patient fill the urinary bladder.
    d. Perform amniocentesis.

105. Where are fetal teratomas most commonly located?
    a. face
    b. neck
    c. sacrococcygeal region
    d. mediastinum

1026   CME Application

106. A patient presents with right-upper-quadrant discomfort, low back pain, and an extremely elevated CA-125. Of the choices listed, which is the most likely cause of the discomfort?
    a. normal liver
    b. perihepatitis
    c. liver abscess
    d. metastatic liver disease

107. The fetal biophysical profile score that indicates that all sonographic parameters are normal is:
    a. 6
    b. 8
    c. 10
    d. 12

108. Where in the placenta does fetal–maternal metabolic exchange occur?
    a. decidua
    b. villi
    c. cotyledons
    d. lobes

109. Which of the following may cause endometriosis?
    a. retrograde menses
    b. infertility
    c. obesity
    d. decreased levels of estrogen

110. When can the dominant ovarian follicle be identified sonographically in an infertility patient?
   a. days 3–5
   b. days 5–7
   c. days 7–9
   d. days 9–10

111. Which abbreviation refers to the procedure whereby an egg is placed in the fallopian tube after fertilization in a Petri dish?
   a. ART
   b. ZIFT
   c. GIFT
   d. IVF

112. Which of the following is a method of quantifying the potential for the ultrasonic heating of human tissue?
   a. thermal index
   b. acoustic output
   c. mechanical index
   d. spatial resolution

113. Doppler waveforms obtained from an artery supplying an intracranial arteriovenous malformation will exhibit:
   a. absent diastolic flow
   b. decreased velocities
   c. triphasic flow
   d. a low pulsatility index

1028   CME Application

114. The ovaries are never visualized in the:
    a. adnexa
    b. anterior cul-de-sac
    c. ovarian fossa
    d. posterior cul-de-sac

115. How early can endovaginal ultrasound identify a gestational sac within the uterine cavity?
    a. 3.5 menstrual weeks
    b. 5.0 menstrual weeks
    c. 5.5 menstrual weeks
    d. 4.5 menstrual weeks

116. n intrauterine gestation composed completely of multisized hydropic villi is called a/an:
    b. hydatidiform mole
    c. a nual pregnancy
    d. hy bryonic pregnancy
        ic degeneration of placenta

117. In what
    a. from ther should the binocular distance be measured?
    b. from the er margin to the inner margin of a single orbit
    c. from the in margin of one orbit to the outer margin of the other orbit
    d. from the out argin of one orbit to the inner margin of the other orbit
        s of one orbit to the outer lens of the other orbit

118. What is the term for adhesions within the endometrial cavity?
    a. polyps
    b. mucosa
    c. adenomyosis
    d. synechiae

119. What endometrial thickness measurement is considered normal in postmenopausal patients receiving unopposed estrogen as hormone replacement therapy?
    a. ≤10 mm
    b. ≤8 mm
    c. ≤6 mm
    d. ≤4 mm

120. Which of the following Doppler findings may be associated with symmetric intrauterine growth restriction (IUGR)?
    a. low-resistance middle cerebral artery
    b. low-resistance umbilical artery
    c. low-resistance ductus venosus
    d. low-resistance renal artery

SCORECARDS CROSS-REFERENCED TO THE ARDMS EXAM CONTENT OUTLINE

Note: For your convenience, <u>ScoreCards</u> questions are arranged according to the task-related topics and subtopics of the ARDMS exam content outline (see www.ardms.org).

ANATOMY AND PHYSIOLOGY

Normal Anatomy and Physiology—GYN, 1, 5, 21, 23, 24, 25, 31, 34, 89, 91, 170, 171, 176, 177, 312, 313, 314, 315, 322, 323, 324, 326, 327, 328, 329, 330, 331, 332, 333, 334, 336, 337, 338, 339, 340, 341, 342, 343, 344, 345, 346, 347, 348, 349, 350, 351, 352, 353, 361, 362, 363, 364, 371, 372, 373, 374, 375, 376, 377, 378, 379, 380, 381, 382, 383, 384, 385, 386, 387, 388, 389, 390, 391, 392, 396, 398, 399, 400, 401, 402, 403, 404, 405, 406, 407, 408, 410, 411, 412, 413, 414, 415, 416, 417, 420, 421, 422, 423, 424, 425, 426, 427, 428, 429, 430, 431, 432, 433, 434, 435, 436, 437, 440, 441, 442, 449, 450, 451, 452, 453, 457, 470, 471, 472, 476, 481, 484

Normal Anatomy and Physiology—OB, 1, 2, 3, 4, 5, 7, 8, 9, 10, 11, 12, 14, 15, 16, 17, 18, 19, 20, 21, 22, 41, 42, 44, 45, 46, 47, 48, 49, 50, 51, 52, 53, 54, 55, 56, 57, 58, 59, 60, 61, 62, 63, 64, 65, 66, 67, 68, 69, 70, 71, 73, 74, 75, 76, 80, 81, 82, 85, 86, 87, 88, 89, 90, 91, 92, 93, 94, 95, 96, 97, 98, 99, 100, 101, 102, 103, 104, 105, 106, 107, 108, 109, 110, 111, 113, 114, 116, 117, 118, 119, 120, 122, 126, 127, 132, 134, 137, 144, 145, 146, 148, 151, 152, 155, 156, 158, 164, 165, 169, 170, 172, 173, 174, 178, 179, 180, 181, 183, 184, 185, 200, 201, 207, 211, 212, 215, 222, 223, 224, 225, 226, 227,

228, 230, 232, 233, 235, 236, 239, 246, 247, 248, 249, 250, 251, 255, 271, 272, 273, 274, 275, 276, 277, 278, 279, 280, 281, 282, 283, 284, 286, 287, 289, 290, 291, 295, 299, 304, 307, 318, 319, 320, 369, 384, 385, 386, 419

PATHOLOGY

Abnormal Physiology and Perfusion—GYN, 23, 24, 175, 311, 312, 313, 314, 315, 321, 322, 323, 324, 336, 350, 378, 380, 381, 382, 392, 396, 407, 408, 409, 410, 411, 412, 413, 414, 415, 416, 417, 418, 419, 420, 421, 422, 423, 424, 425, 426, 427, 428, 429, 430, 431, 432, 433, 434, 435, 436, 437, 438, 439, 440, 441, 442, 449, 450, 451, 452, 454, 455, 456, 457, 474, 476

Abnormal Physiology and Perfusion—OB, 168, 169, 175, 176, 311, 438, 439, 440, 454, 455, 474

Congenital Anomalies, 6, 9, 10, 11, 14, 26, 27, 29, 30, 31, 32, 33, 34, 35, 36, 37, 38, 39, 64, 65, 66, 82, 84, 95, 97, 98, 101, 102, 104, 130, 132, 134, 137, 140, 141, 142, 143, 147, 149, 150, 153, 154, 157, 158, 162, 165, 170, 172, 173, 174, 183, 186, 187, 193, 194, 195, 196, 197, 198, 199, 200, 201, 202, 204, 205, 206, 207, 208, 209, 210, 211, 212, 213, 214, 216, 217, 218, 219, 220, 221, 222, 223, 224, 225, 226, 227, 228, 229, 230, 231, 232, 233, 234, 235, 236, 237, 238, 239, 240, 241, 242, 243, 244, 245, 246, 247, 248, 249, 250, 251, 252, 253, 254, 255, 256, 257, 258, 259, 260, 261, 262, 263, 264, 265, 266, 267, 268, 269, 270, 271, 272, 273, 274, 275, 276, 277, 278, 279, 280, 281, 282, 283, 284, 285, 286, 287, 288, 289, 290, 291, 293, 294, 295, 296, 299, 300, 301, 302, 303, 304, 305, 306, 307, 308, 309, 310, 314, 315, 316, 317, 318, 319, 320, 325, 383, 384, 385, 386, 451, 455

Placental Abnormalities, 28, 90, 92, 96, 98, 106, 107, 108, 109, 110, 111, 112, 114, 119, 120, 168, 473

PROTOCOLS

Clinical Standards and Guidelines, 13, 31, 34, 36, 83, 84, 106, 109, 111, 122, 158, 159, 160, 161, 162, 163, 166, 167, 186, 187, 213, 214, 236, 245, 295, 316, 317, 327, 328, 329, 331, 359, 360, 365, 366, 367, 368, 369, 370, 382, 389, 391, 393, 394, 395, 396, 397, 408, 409, 410, 414, 421, 424, 431, 432, 433, 434, 436, 440, 442, 445, 446, 449, 450, 451, 452, 456, 457, 458, 459, 460, 461, 462, 463, 464, 465, 466, 467, 468, 469, 473, 474, 476, 477, 478, 480, 482, 486, 487, 494

Measurement Techniques—GYN, 164, 171, 177, 326, 328, 332, 335, 387, 388, 402, 403, 447, 448, 449, 459, 481

Measurement Techniques—OB, 2, 8, 11, 12, 16, 40, 43, 44, 53, 72, 77, 78, 79, 121, 123, 124, 125, 126, 127, 128, 129, 130, 131, 132, 133, 134, 135, 136, 137, 138, 139, 140, 174, 178, 179, 180, 181, 182, 183, 199, 211, 222, 285, 296, 297, 298, 306

PHYSICS AND INSTRUMENTATION

Hemodynamics—GYN, 114, 115, 203, 352, 353, 354, 355, 356, 357, 358, 432, 443

Hemodynamics—OB, 30, 71, 102, 143, 292, 293, 294, 358, 490

Imaging Instruments, 30, 82, 102, 292, 389, 444, 475, 479, 483, 484, 485, 486, 487, 488, 489, 490, 491, 492, 493, 495

TREATMENT

Sonographer Role in Procedures, 157, 184, 185, 188, 189, 190, 191, 192, 393, 409